Benchmarking in Health Care

A Collaborative Approach

by
Robert G. Gift
and
Doug Mosel

AHA books are published by
American Hospital Publishing, Inc.,
an American Hospital Association company

The views expressed in this publication are strictly those of the authors and do not necessarily represent official positions of the American Hospital Association.

Library of Congress Cataloging-in-Publication Data

Gift, Robert G.
    Benchmarking in health care : a collaborative approach / Robert G.
Gift, Doug Mosel.
      p.   cm.
    Includes bibliographical references.
    ISBN 1-55648-125-X (pbk.)
    1. Health services administration. 2. Benchmarking (Management).
I. Mosel, Doug.   II. Title.
    [DNLM: 1. Delivery of Health Care—organization & administration—
United States. 2. Quality of Health Care—organization &
administration—United States. W 84 AA1 G36b 1994]
DNLM/DLC
for Library of Congress   94-22781
                                               CIP

Catalog no. 169107

©1994 by American Hospital Publishing, Inc.,
an American Hospital Association company

Printed in the USA

Text set in Goudy
2.5M—11/94—0384

Audrey Kaufman, Acquisitions and Development Editor
Nancy Charpentier, Production Editor
Peggy DuMais, Production Coordinator
Cheryl Kusek, Cover Designer
Marcia Bottoms, Books Division Assistant Director
Brian Schenk, Books Division Director

Contents

List of Figures

About the Authors

Robert G. Gift, MS, is vice-president, quality and productivity improvement, for the Catholic Health Corporation (CHC) in Omaha, Nebraska. He is responsible for the design, development, and initiation of the corporation's approach to total quality management; the analysis and design of systems that enhance service delivery while reducing costs; and the development of methodologies for detailed analysis of systemwide productivity and quality issues.

Before joining CHC, Mr. Gift worked as an independent consultant, conducting projects in planning, financial modeling, and operations improvement. He has served in several administrative management positions, both inside and outside of CHC. He began his health care career as a management engineer in an 1,100-bed medical teaching facility.

Mr. Gift holds a bachelor's degree in industrial engineering and a master's degree in operations research, both from the University of Pittsburgh. He has completed additional course work in public health and business administration.

Mr. Gift has authored several articles on quality improvement, productivity management, and organizational performance. In addition, he has delivered numerous presentations on quality management topics, cost strategies, and planning for operational improvements.

Doug Mosel, MS, teaches and advises in health care quality management and organizational transformation. He is interested in applied systems thinking and chaos/change theory, collaboration and teamwork, and benchmarking. Until June 1994, he served as director of CQI education for VHA Tri-State, Inc., in Indianapolis, where he developed the nationally recognized program of the Institute for CQI Education for 21 member hospitals. He has developed and taught institute courses in quality management and he has published articles on quality and collaboration in health care.

Mr. Mosel has consulted and presented nationally and internationally in health care management. Before joining VHA Tri-State in 1991, he served as quality coach at Memorial Hospital and Health System in South Bend, Indiana, where he assisted in the development and implementation of Memorial's Quality Through People process and led the quality and organization development department. Mr. Mosel has taught both graduates and under-graduates at the university level and was a principal in his own consulting practice for seven years before becoming part of the Memorial team in 1985.

Mr. Mosel earned his bachelor's degree in education and theology at Concordia, River Forest, Illinois, and his master's in education and counseling at Indiana University in Bloomington. He completed professional development programs in training and organizational development with NTL Institute and University Associates.

Foreword

From Robert C. Camp, PhD, PE (Manager, Benchmarking Competency, Xerox Corporation)

The quality improvement tool known in business as benchmarking is beginning to take hold throughout various segments of U.S. economy and around the globe. From its early origins in the manufacturing sector, benchmarking has spilled over into the service arena and is reaching into the nonprofit sector (most notably health care), the government, and slowly into education. This trend, also identified in Europe, Asia Pacific, and South America, probably is occurring, no doubt, simply because it works. Unlike other improvement activities of the past, benchmarking capitalizes on the principle of learning from others: If best (or better) practices are determined to exist elsewhere, then the opportunity is presented to understand them and then adapt them creatively to improve current practices.

Although this principle may be understood in its concept, the reality is that organizations need to have the basic benchmarking approach translated into their specific settings. It is commendable, therefore, that health care planners and quality managers are doing just that and furthermore are developing case history examples of actual application.

In fact, of all segments of the economy, the health care profession perhaps has been the fastest learner and implementer of benchmarking. That too is commendable.

But perhaps most helpful is the availability of texts that translate benchmarking concepts into the language, setting, and culture of the profession. In this book Gift and Mosel accomplish that purpose and, as indicated by the title, position the book appropriately within health care so that practitioners learn collaboratively to effect breakthrough improvement.

I believe *Benchmarking in Health Care* to be an excellent addition to the art and science of benchmarking. I welcome new perspectives and adaptations of this important quality tool and warmly recommend it to the reader.

From Philip A. Newbold (President and CEO, Memorial Hospital)

The command-and-control style of management is dead. Replacing this 1960s top-down philosophy is one of collaboration and cooperation, where knowledge and power are shared among the many rather than hoarded by an elite few. This change, increasingly prominent in health care, has its origins in the industrial sector, where the notion that a few highly placed individuals within organizations know best or could possibly manage all complexities of multiple operations has been abandoned in favor of a new spirit of working with a team focus.

Benchmarking in Health Care: A Collaborative Approach presents a model based on this new spirit of working collaboratively, learning from others, and realizing dramatic – or breakthrough – improvements in all health care practices, processes, and systems. At its roots benchmarking is about learning from others, first by analyzing key processes of operations and then searching within and outside an industry or professional area for the best demonstrated practices.

A chief force that will propel health care providers into embracing benchmarking more aggressively is the move from fee-for-service medicine toward prepayment or capitation. This shift from an acute care focus to one of prevention for and accountability to the health status of a defined population will lead providers to examine strategies for breakthrough improvements. With these changes comes the press for continuous quality improvement in services as well as better clinical outcomes, lower health care costs, and greater accessibility to effective health care for all segments of the population.

It is extremely liberating to be able to search the entire industrial and health care landscape for new models, methodologies, and tools to meet the challenges that confront the nation's health care system. It also is frightening to think of abandoning traditional ways of delivering and financing health care under the shift to prepayment for services. Yet the learning mind-set that benchmarking reinforces is what will lead providers to look to the expertise of others – health care and non-health care top performers – from whom they can learn new approaches. Critical to this effort are formal and informal networks and alliances built around leaders' visions for seeking rapid improvements in outcomes.

The origins of benchmarking, I believe, belong under the umbrella of continuous quality improvement, where the power of teams and team-based learning is one of the most liberating and self-empowering aspects of the quality improvement movement in U.S. health care. In learning to harness the power of "groupthink" as they seek to improve processes and clinical outcomes, leaders embrace a new style of doing health care, essentially by empowering individuals at every level of each organization. Benchmarking, then, is a vehicle that can help providers move beyond incremental improvements seen over the past five years with CQI to high-speed breakthroughs in key processes and performance.

One of the most significant examples of breakthrough is the movement toward work redesign and reengineering. Another is the patient-focused care movement—organizing care around the needs, expectations, and requirements of patients—which has yielded tremendous success to a number of hospitals around the country. Secondary benefits of both movements accrue to staff who through working with teams enjoy more access to technology and training opportunities and, ultimately, job expansion and enrichment. Both patients and staff benefit as services are brought closer to the bedside (bedside admissions, for example). Breakthroughs will continue as health care processes and delivery systems are reengineered, starting first with the more expensive high-technology inpatient care and extending through ambulatory and community-based care.

Drawing on their extensive experience in benchmarking, the authors make a compelling case for the models and concepts of this discipline as it is applied in health care. They also make it clear that old models based on competition must give way to collaborative models based on information exchange. As hospitals evolve into "wholistic" health care systems in their communities, lessons learned and strategies and models used for benchmarking become applicable in a range of new ways. Whether the health care problem to be solved arises at a community, organizational, systems, or individual level the philosophy, tools, and methods described here can help toward solution.

Years from now when they look back at the 1990s, providers will appreciate how far their thinking and approach to change management and problem solving have come. *Benchmarking in Health Care* will be recognized as one of those important books that helped shape this new thinking.

Preface

"Re-create yourself, or die" might be the dictum for health care organizations as they prepare for the 21st century. This transformation requires changes of unprecedented scope and magnitude on the part of organizations to develop their capacity to assume responsibility for the health status of the communities they serve. Services must be provided faster, at less cost, and with better results. This means that organizational work processes must be improved and structures changed at near-blinding speed; then improved and changed again, with virtually no period of stability. For most health care organizations, this means improvement and change in breakthrough proportions.

To achieve transformation of this magnitude, organizations must create cultures that facilitate rapid change in the midst of a chaotic and unpredictable health care environment. Therefore, leaders face a formidable challenge, not the least of which is to close the gap quickly between current knowledge and new learning needed to accomplish these unprecedented changes. Furthermore, a growing body of evidence demonstrates that old ways of learning are no longer adequate.

So, health care providers benchmark to learn how to perform the work of health care delivery in ways to achieve breakthrough results — faster, simpler, less costly, more efficiently, and matched more consistently to customer requirements. This is the immediate reason for benchmarking. The longer view is that each experience enhances the organization's capacity for learning. Each benchmarking team is like a neuron with a direct connection to the organization's collective brain, transmitting not only lessons learned about work processes, but about learning itself. From this standpoint, even a benchmarking project that fails to achieve process performance goals provides a rich opportunity to enhance the learning skills of team members, managers, and leaders.

The future for health care organizations requires more cooperation and coordination among service providers because no single organization can shoulder the full responsibility for improving the health status of a community. This thinking reflects the understanding among providers that each one is part of a larger whole and as such is dependent on other providers across the full continuum of care. Such shared responsibility requires collaborative learning so as to provide services effectively and with a minimum of duplication and waste. That learning must take place in a cooperative arena for all to benefit.

Purpose of This Book

This book was written in response to the need for a model to bridge the above-mentioned learning gap collaboratively. Following discussions with health care executives and quality professionals, we determined that the book should dispel some of the mystique surrounding benchmarking which, like so many new approaches, resides in the domain of a few specialists or consultants. The model presented builds on health care organizations' experience with continuous quality improvement. Therefore, we designed the internal and external phases of the benchmarking approach around Shewhart's plan-do-study-act cycle. Both phases incorporate tools known to those involved with quality improvement efforts.

In addition to building on existing knowledge and experience, we saw a need for an approach that advocates the value of collaboration on the part of multiple organizations. Three reasons underlie this decision: First, health care organizations have far more experience with competition than with cooperation. Collaborative benchmarking, which provides a powerful opportunity to learn the mutual benefits of working together, offers health care leaders a relatively low-risk practicum in which to enhance their skills at cooperation. Second, a collaborative benchmarking project is dramatically more cost-effective for each participating organization—a fraction of what one provider would spend in an independent effort. Finally, organizational learning, the fundamental reason for benchmarking, is conditioned on collaboration and is an underlying assumption throughout this book.

Audience

Benchmarking in Health Care was developed for use by health care executives, quality professionals (planners and managers, for example), and benchmarking practitioners. The book provides leadership teams with rationale for applying benchmarking in health care organizations, including benefits to providers. Quality professionals are presented detailed steps of an approach they may wish to adapt into their quality improvement toolbox. For example, they can use the materials for training new benchmarking teams. Experienced benchmarking practitioners will find in the book alternative methodology and a solid reference resource.

Overview of the Book

This book is presented in three sections. Part one, An Introduction to Benchmarking, contains two chapters. Chapter 1 defines and explores benchmarking as a methodology for breakthrough improvement in health care delivery. Chapter 2 discusses the rationale for applying benchmarking in health care organizations.

Part two, The Collaborative Benchmarking Model, details the progression of activities that comprise the model. Chapter 3 gives an overview of the four phases in the collaborative project. Chapter 4 focuses on selecting the benchmarking project. Chapter 5 discusses the steps required to establish the collaborative. Chapter 6 describes procedures for conducting the project within a collaborative. Chapter 7 details procedures involved in conducting the project with partners outside the collaborative. Chapter 8 reviews methods for managing a benchmarking team, an important contributor to overall success of the collaborative effort.

Part three, made up of chapter 9, identifies pitfalls to avoid in using the model. In addition to describing some of the challenges that confront the collaborative, it provides some speculation on the future application of benchmarking within the health care sector.

Acknowledgments

We are indebted to many organizations and individuals without whose support, encouragement, and assistance this work could not have been created. We recognize the Healthcare Forum, its Team Quality members (Keith McCandless, Stefanie Fenton, and Tracy Conway), and the members of its Quality Improvement Networks for providing the stimulus for launching this effort. They helped us identify the need for adapting a model for use by health care organizations.

We thank the Catholic Health Corporation for unflagging support in developing the collaborative model for benchmarking. The Management Staff of the organization, particularly A. Diane Moeller (chief executive officer) and Eleanor G. Claus (president, Midwest/Western Division), repeatedly demonstrated two of the organization's core values — collaboration and risk/trust — in allowing us to experiment with this approach. Special thanks go to all those involved with the Worker's Compensation Benchmarking Project — the Design Team, the Steering Committee, and the Facility Benchmarking Teams — for their efforts in providing a laboratory in which to incubate the model. The Quality & Productivity Improvement Staff warrant particular recognition for their encouragement, support, and patience with the demands during development of this project. We hope it will be a worthwhile contribution to their benchmarking endeavors.

We appreciate the support of colleagues in VHA Tri-State, Inc. for their encouragement and interest in benchmarking and this project. We hope this work is helpful to benchmarkers there.

We recognize the contribution of Bruce E. Hopkins, president, Aquila Management, for his encouragement and support. His suggestions, based on a reading of the manuscript, led to improvements in the final text.

Audrey Kaufman, acquisitions and development editor, American Hospital Publishing, Inc., provided large doses of guidance and assistance to two novices in their initial foray into writing a book. She worked with us cooperatively to overcome complexities imposed by distance, travel schedules, and our "day jobs." The book reflects her insightful comments and considerable editorial talent.

Our friends and families deserve our thanks for their tolerance during our writing and editing of this book, and for their undaunting belief in us and in the value of this effort. Last, we express gratitude to those who have traveled the benchmarking trail before us. Without their courage, help, and guidance, this approach and subsequent book could not have been developed.

We hope this book contributes to the practice of benchmarking in health care organizations. We hope it helps them build their capacities for collaboration, learning, and breakthrough.

Part One

An Introduction to Benchmarking

THE FAR SIDE   By GARY LARSON

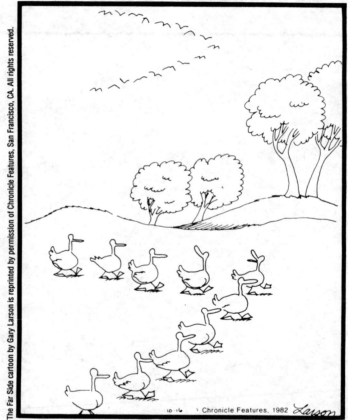

"Say ... Look what THEY'RE doing."

Chapter One

What Is Benchmarking?

In quality management, the term benchmark has been used to designate the best designs or best practices.[1] [It has also been called] . . . stealing shamelessly[2] [and] . . . learning from others.[3]

Introduction

Benchmarking has rapidly become a major phenomenon in health care. The term is used widely, although its meaning varies from one setting to another and its application lacks consistency.

This chapter describes what benchmarking is, its origins in industry, and its adaptation to the health care arena. The chapter also describes three types of benchmarking and offers an approach that is appropriate for health care providers. Finally, those elements that enhance or impede a benchmarking project—referred to in this book as prerequisites and accelerators—are examined as they relate to successful implementation.

Industrial Roots

Like continuous quality improvement, benchmarking originated in an industrial setting. Xerox Corporation and Robert Camp, its manager of benchmarking competency, are recognized pioneers of benchmarking in the United States. Xerox formally defined *benchmarking* as "the continuous process of measuring products, services, and practices against the toughest competitors or those companies recognized as industry leaders."[4] Camp, acknowledged benchmarking guru, defines the term briefly as "finding and implementing best practices."[5]

Another acknowledged leader in the application of benchmarking is AT&T, where the practice has been an acknowledged fundamental business priority. The AT&T definition emphasizes the study of processes and their integration into organizational operations: "Benchmarking is the process by which you measure the operational performance of the 'Best in Class' performers, then determine how that performance is achieved and how it best can be transferred into your operations, and once having done this then integrating this opportunity into your business planning, strategies, plans, budgets, etc. for improvement and continual monitoring for new emerging Benchmarks."[6]

Health Care Beginnings

A small number of health care organizations have made thoughtful and successful beginnings in benchmarking, which The SunHealth Alliance defines as "a . . . process for identifying specifications for best results, ways to measure them, and work methods and practices that assure the specs are met consistently."[7] Catholic Health Corporation calls benchmarking "the continual discipline of measuring our results, comparing those results with others, learning how those results are achieved, and applying those lessons for breakthrough improvement."[8] Voluntary Hospitals of America, Inc., borrowing from Camp, defines it as "the process of finding and implementing best practices."[9]

Common Characteristics

Five elements are common to these definitions and to others used throughout health care and other settings.

1. *Benchmarking is understood to be a process, a structured approach, or a discipline.* In other words, it is a systematic approach that makes use of appropriate methods and tools.
2. *The process is continuous or ongoing.* It is utilized regularly, rather than as a one-time activity.
3. *Benchmarking involves measuring, evaluating, and comparing both results and the processes that produce the results.* The practice is data driven.
4. *Benchmarking focuses on best results and best practices.* The intent is to study and adapt the leading practices, those that produce "benchmark" results.
5. *The goal of the benchmarking study is improvement to at least the level of best-in-class.* Where possible, the goal is to surpass that level of performance.

The following three elements, although not explicitly included in many of the definitions, are considered fundamental to successful benchmarking:

1. *Focusing on key products, services, or processes.* Leaders in the practice of benchmarking, such as Xerox, have identified those business processes that are of strategic importance to their success. Leading health care organizations also are beginning to adopt core processes as the focus of their benchmarking efforts.
2. *Learning from others.* Relatively few definitions of benchmarking explicitly identify learning from others as basic to the practice. Nonetheless, adopting the orientation of "learner" is essential to success.

3. *Applying what has been learned.* Although no one denies that best practices must be adapted to fit specific organizations, a surprising number of definitions fail to incorporate this critical concept. Part of every benchmarking project must be the determination of *how to apply* what is learned.

In addition to the above benchmarking building blocks drawn from others, the following two should be added as crucial to health care practice:

1. *Improving patient care practices.* The fundamental purpose of health care benchmarking is to improve health care delivery. Thus, it is not sufficient to focus efforts primarily on administrative or support processes.
2. *Building healthier communities.* The ultimate reason for a health care organization to benchmark the processes of care delivery is to make people healthier, *not* to increase market share. Only this higher purpose of community service will sustain improvement efforts throughout the chaos of health care reform.

A Definition for the Health Care Setting

Webster's defines *benchmark* only as a noun — a mark, standard, or reference point. The term is commonly used, however, as both noun (a target performance level) and verb (to study and adapt the processes that produce the target performance). Because it refers to a mark on a *stationary* object, the dictionary definition is inadequate for the purposes of this book; the target performances sought in health care benchmarking are *dynamic*. Thus, the authors have adapted the following definition:

> Health care benchmarking is the continual and collaborative discipline of measuring and comparing the results of key work processes with those of the best performers. It is learning how to adapt these best practices to achieve breakthrough process improvements and build healthier communities.

Implications

In health care, benchmarking is understood to be a disciplined approach, not just a technique. Therefore it is continual, "repeated regularly and frequently; recurring often."[10] Also, it is focused on those outcomes and related core processes known to be most important to customers and is understood to be a learning process by which best practices are transferred and adapted to the organization.

Benchmarking is essentially a scientific approach and as such is aligned with the training and practice of clinicians. Collaboration, not competition, is the better way to improve practices and outcomes on behalf of those served. If the purpose of benchmarking is to serve the common good of health care providers and their communities, individual health care organizations will thrive as well.

Three Types of Benchmarking

Practitioners and the growing body of literature in the field generally recognize three types of benchmarking. They are internal, competitive, and functional, as summarized in figure 1-1.

Internal Benchmarking

Even though internal benchmarking offers the least potential for breakthrough improvement, it is a low-risk way to learn and practice the discipline and to achieve uniform results. It can be easily undertaken by quality improvement teams and is the most appropriate form of benchmarking for the institution new to continuous quality improvement (CQI). For example, departments might study on-the-job training practices in other departments within the organization, or clinicians might examine treatment protocols used by colleagues in their practice or specialty. Hopefully, internal benchmarking, a natural for routine use by a hospital system or multisite health care organization, will become standard practice.

Competitive and Functional Benchmarking

Competitive benchmarking and functional benchmarking offer the greatest potential for breakthrough improvement. Robert Ogle, of Johnson & Johnson, asserts that 90 percent of the opportunity for breakthrough improvement results from these external forms of benchmarking.[11] Competitive benchmarking enables the organization to learn from the best practices (for example, surgery scheduling or customer service) within the health care field, regardless of whether they

Figure 1-1. Types of Benchmarking

Type	Definition	Examples
Internal	Best practices within the organization; "internal best"	• Equipment: sterilizer, washer • Same process, different practitioners: surgical procedure, room cleaning, record transcription, therapy • Operations: unit record keeping, transportation, patient registration
Competitive	Best performer in market or in health care; "competitive best"	• Any comparable product, process, or procedure in a similar health care organization
Functional	Cross-industry comparison of the same or analogous process; "best in class"	• Registration or food service in hotels; supplier relations in the auto industry; billing in American Express • Clinical applications of technology: lasers

are performed within the organization or by a competitor. In functional benchmarking, practices that commonly are performed in other industries as well as in health care, such as information processing, customer intake, or technology applications, may be studied with partners outside the health care profession. Taking advantage of competitive or functional benchmarking opportunities requires the most effort and resources and, therefore, the greatest organizational commitment. Further, the success of these approaches depends on availability of a solid base of experience in CQI methods and tools. The health care organization without CQI experience is well advised to learn and practice quality improvement methods as a preparation for benchmarking.

A Recommended Approach for Health Care: Collaboration

Any of the three types of benchmarking as described above can be applied successfully in health care. The authors' experience with CQI in health care demonstrates that the most effective advantage of internal, competitive, or functional benchmarking is achieved through provider collaboration. (See figure 1-2.) Because it is supportive of each type of benchmarking, a collaborative effort lends itself to health care for a number of reasons:

- The industry is made up of common work processes across providers, from patient registration to complex surgical procedures.
- Documentation of practice and outcome variation within these common processes supports the need for, and benefit of, collaboration.
- A collaborative approach to benchmarking conserves resources previously expended on reinventing solutions as individual organizations.
- Collaborative benchmarking is more cost-effective because project costs are shared among all participants. (Specific costs are detailed later in the chapter.)

Figure 1-2. Collaborative Benchmarking

Approach	Search for:	Focus on:
Collaboration through voluntary network of health care providers	1. Best practice in the collaborative 2. Best practice in health care or market 3. Best practice in another industry	• Any comparable product, process, or procedure

- Collaboration serves as an improvement accelerator, speeding up adjustments to the shift from an acute care focus to a vision of healthier communities, with the cooperation among various providers and ancillary organizations.
- This approach shifts from comparing data to comparing and understanding processes critical to effective and efficient health care delivery.
- A collaborative approach benefits all participants mutually and helps to break down the isolation that historically has separated health care organizations. For example, instead of paying external experts to arrive at "solutions" already developed at other organizations, collaboration helps disseminate learning, promotes provider cooperation, and facilitates the learning of a transferable improvement methodology.

Taken together, these reasons suggest that collaboration is the optimal strategy for taking advantage of the powerful discipline of benchmarking in health care.

As already mentioned, a collaborative approach has strong precedent in industry as well as in health care. Camp suggests that benchmarking be ". . . calculated to obtain the cooperation of benchmarking partners. . . . There should be a constant sharing of ideas and debating about how the industry is going to constantly improve itself. . . . Benchmarking should be approached on a partnership basis in which both parties should expect to gain from the information sharing."[12] In *The Benchmarking Book*, Michael J. Spendolini points out the growing practice of forming benchmarking networks or consortia within and across industries as a way of initiating studies and sharing resources.[13]

Prerequisites and Accelerators in Benchmarking Success

Benchmarking, as defined earlier, is an ongoing process that measures, evaluates, and compares selected activities against a best-practice target. Two elements can make or break a benchmarking project: prerequisites and accelerators.

Prerequisites

Four prerequisites should be in place before an organization initiates a benchmarking project. These are commitment on the part of leaders, the organization's experience with CQI, organizational preparation, and identification of key processes.

Leadership Commitment

As with CQI, benchmarking requires the consistent, long-term commitment of organizational leadership. That commitment must be three-dimensional in intent. It should meet and exceed the needs of all customers who depend on the organization; focus organizational attention on the system of work processes that serve customers; and transform that system and its component processes.

Leadership commitment is a challenging prerequisite, given the tendency of health care leaders to seek quick fixes in an atmosphere that demands immediate breakthrough improvements. The quality of commitment is further complicated by leaders who historically have misconstrued *any* comparison with another organization as benchmarking.

CQI Experience

Benchmarking is a process that uses most of the same tools and techniques used in continuous quality improvement, or total quality management (TQM). Yet benchmarking, like TQM and CQI, is much more than technique; it is a continuous practice. Ogle (Johnson & Johnson) made the observation that best-in-class is a moving target, requiring that benchmarking be an ongoing activity.[14] It is also a discipline and, AT&T suggests, ". . . there are several disciplines you must know and practice before acceptable results are produced."[15] These disciplines involve not only learning the process, but developing the support and patience necessary for benchmarking to succeed.

As indicated earlier, benchmarking represents a new way, a paradigm shift. Says Camp: "Benchmarking is a way to manage, not an added management task. It is not an attempt to simply copy or transport someone else's 'best practice' to a hospital department, but a process of combining other organizations' best practices with yours to achieve optimal effectiveness given your department's uniquenesses."[16] In effect, Camp describes benchmarking as an experiential management activity.

The focus on experience with CQI principles, methods, and tools, then, is a prerequisite to optimal use of this potent means to breakthrough improvements. Continuous quality improvement reaffirms customers as the reason behind improvement efforts, processes as the target of those efforts, and the scientific method as the vehicle through which significant improvement occurs. If benchmarking is to be utilized systematically and proactively, rather than sporadically and reactively, it must occur within a management culture that understands and supports its use through experiential application. Quality management provides a structure for identifying and prioritizing opportunities for improvement, which is a key objective of benchmarking studies. The CQI structure also incorporates implementation follow-through and improvements monitoring, both of which are as critical in benchmarking as they are in CQI.

Organizational Preparation

Even an organization that has considerable CQI experience needs to prepare its management team for a benchmarking project and provide the framework to ensure success. Toward this end, benchmarking should be introduced to senior managers first, both to gain their support and to prepare them to use and teach the process. Given the provider tendency for short-term fascination with the latest methodologies, it is advisable to introduce benchmarking as a strategic component or an extension of CQI, rather than as a "new program."

Organizational preparation is important not only for the success of the benchmarking project, but for the change implicit in seeking breakthrough improvement. Indeed, the ultimate test of benchmarking is *whether* things change: "A good way to tell the difference between companies that merely pay lip service to the concept [of change] and those that actually practice it is to look for evidence of change – the end point of the benchmarking process. It's no coincidence that avid benchmarkers undergo radical operational and organizational changes."[17]

Identification of Key Processes

Key processes, referred to by the Joint Commission on Accreditation of Healthcare Organizations (JCAHO) as "important functions," are those essential activities that must be performed optimally to meet customers' needs. These key processes (or functions) comprise the whole system which in health care is known as a health care organization. Patient admissions, testing, and surgery, for example, are three key processes of the larger system.

Identifying key processes is an important benchmarking prerequisite for several reasons. Applying the Pareto principle, key processes represent the "critical few" opportunities for break-through improvement. Once an important function has been singled out, the benchmarking effort has a focus, so that the leadership team or quality council finds it easier to prioritize products, services, or processes to benchmark.

Key process identification helps the team form a framework for managing the benchmarking effort. Parkview Episcopal Medical Center (Pueblo, Colorado) assigns a coordinating committee to each of their key processes: same-day surgery and operating room; admissions/billing/discharge; dietary services; clinical results reporting; environmental services; and clinical care – pneumonia, cardiac cath lab; cardiac surgery; stroke; schizophrenia; total hip surgery; C-sections. For example, the coordinating committee for clinical care provides direction for improvement teams working on pneumonia, stroke, total hip replacement, and so forth.

Using key processes to build a framework helps ensure a cohesive benchmarking effort. This avoids any suboptimization that can occur if disproportionate attention is called to any one process under scrutiny. Figure 1-3 (developed by Palto Alto Medical Foundation and Shaw Resources) shows how the Palo Alto Medical Foundation maintains this interrelatedness by using a flowchart to display key processes as components of a larger system.

Finally, key process identification helps streamline costs. Benchmarking is resource-intensive, with external studies requiring from 6 to 10 times the investment needed for an internal quality improvement team. As pressure mounts to reduce costs, quality councils will have to apply the Pareto principle to select

Figure 1-3. QI Flowchart Maps a Patient Pathway

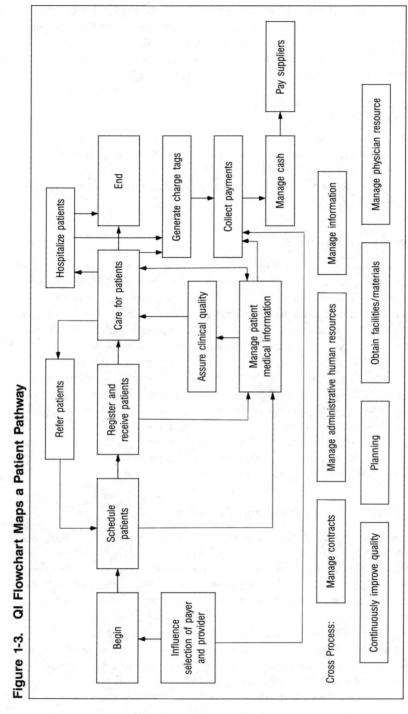

Copyright Palo Alto Medical Foundation, Palo Alto, CA, and Shaw Resources, Cupertino, CA. Used with permission.

the critical few processes in which to invest scarce resources. Those selected must have the greatest impact on patients, the community, and the organization in terms of critical outcome areas such as health status, cost, or time. Once identified, key processes offer a ready-made framework for determining which processes, when improved, will create the most leverage.

Accelerators

Although the four prerequisites delineated contribute much to a project's success, they do not ensure optimal benchmarking. Any one of several variables also must be in place to accelerate the strategy. Three of these accelerators—learning capacity, knowledge of customers and processes, and resource availability—are described below.

Capacity for Learning

A health care organization achieves breakthrough improvements in processes in direct proportion to its development as a learning organization. Learning from others is at the heart of the benchmarking process, but health care providers, although fast learners, have been slow to transfer practices learned from those outside health care. Within the field, and particularly within defined markets, a competitive stance blocks many opportunities for learning.

In writing on the conditions necessary for effective learning, systems thinking expert Stefanie Spear, of In Care, says that developing ". . . a learning organization requires mastery of a collaborative learning process."[18] A guiding principle of the process is the understanding of *systemness*. "How can we do this," poses Spear, "in a way that serves equally both those in the enterprise *and* those in the community, rather than serving one at the expense of the other?"[19] The answer may lie in organizational capacity for learning, which can accelerate or retard the effectiveness of benchmarking.

Knowledge of Customers and Processes

In health care generally, lack of knowledge about customers and care processes significantly limits the potential effectiveness of benchmarking. This knowledge deficit is exacerbated by inadequate measurement strategies and information systems, a deficit so severe that a report by Lisa O'Rourke and Barry Bader calls it "healthcare's Achilles heel: The field is sadly lacking in the kind of automated information systems that managing for quality demands."[20]

Most providers still depend primarily on retrospective satisfaction surveys or complaint summaries for knowledge about patient expectations. A few use more advanced strategies, such as focus groups or patient representatives, to gather information. Although clinical assessments and high-technology diagnostic services yield sophisticated care profiles, that information is generally event-focused and reactive, that is, generated only in response to illness or injury.

Within individual organizations, knowledge of internal processes and performance variations is also limited. Instead of focusing on which processes lead to which outcomes and critical variables in those processes, leaders are preoccupied with outcomes driven by financial, productivity, and regulatory mandates. One reason, according to O'Rourke and Bader, is that hospitals have invested only 3–4 percent of expenses in information systems. By contrast, "Almost any other sophisticated industry is investing six to eight percent of its expenses in information systems."[21] Consequently, gathering data on the performance of most key health care processes requires special studies. Long-term success with benchmarking will require providers to redirect substantial investment dollars into measurement strategies and information systems that are attuned to the needs of customers as well as the processes that serve them. Otherwise, learning for breakthrough improvements will be retarded rather than accelerated.

Resource Availability

Again, benchmarking is a resource-intensive activity. According to the International Benchmarking Clearinghouse of the American Productivity and Quality Center, direct costs of an external benchmarking study can range from $30,000 to $60,000; a project can cost as much as $100,000. As already suggested, a collaborative approach to benchmarking can significantly reduce these costs for participating organizations.

Cost breakdowns vary among institutions, but four key cost areas are as follows:

1. *Training:* Involves educating team members, leaders, and facilitators in benchmarking methods and team management
2. *Direct project costs:* Include data-collection studies, travel, investment in improvements, consultants
3. *Information systems:* Provide support functions for data gathering, analysis, and dissemination for continuous benchmarking
4. *Salaries:* Provide compensation and other incentives for benchmarking team

Given the current state of knowledge about quality and information systems, it is likely that initial investment in benchmarking will be hefty. The collaborative approach proposed in this book spreads this investment across participating organizations that are bound by scarce resources and pressure to reduce costs. Sharing the costs of a project thus enhances resource availability and utilization to accelerate efforts.

Summary

Benchmarking is a powerful and accessible tool for achieving breakthrough performance in key processes, in both patient care and support areas. Benchmarking both promotes and depends on the learning orientation of an organization. A collaborative approach is economical, permitting more organizations to take full advantage of the potential effects of successful benchmarking, one of which is improved cooperation among health care providers. Only through meeting the prerequisites (leadership commitment, CQI experience, preparation, and key process identification), as well as the accelerators (capacity to learn, knowledge of customers and processes, and resource availability) can an organization achieve this end.

Putting These Ideas to Work

Objective

Assess the readiness of your organization to make optimal use of benchmarking.

Approach

With your leadership team or quality council, complete the benchmarking readiness assessment (figure 1-4), study the decision/action flowchart (figure 1-5), discuss implications of the responses, and where indicated take action to enhance your organization's potential to maximize the benefits.

Figure 1-4. Benchmarking Readiness Assessment

Question	Yes	No	Action if "No"
1. Is leadership commitment to benchmarking driven by customers, processes, and transformation?			Develop and implement a plan to increase understanding among leaders.
2. Does senior management understand benchmarking as a strategic component of TQM?			Repeat preceding action.
3. Does the organization have at least three years' experience with TQM?			Accelerate organizational preparation, including experience with TQM.
4. Has the organization identified key processes?			Identify key processes.
5. Does the organization have a well-developed capacity for learning?			Plan and implement a strategy to support organizational learning.
6. Is the organization's knowledge base of customers and processes well established?			Establish an infrastructure and processes required to build this knowledge base.
7. Does senior leadership clearly prioritize resources to support benchmarking?			Step up prioritization of resources allocated for support breakthrough.

Figure 1-5. Decision/Action Flowchart for Benchmarking Readiness

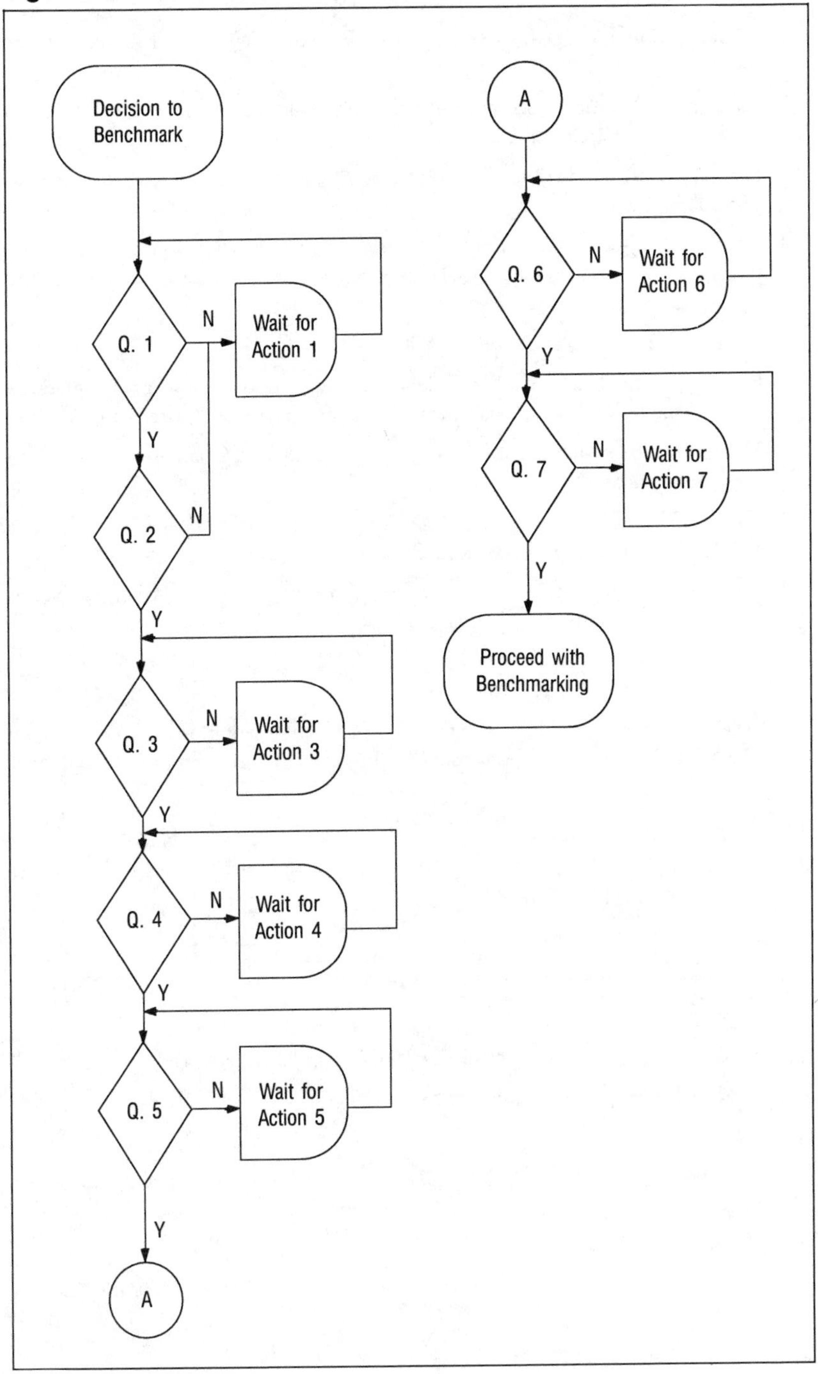

References

1. Juran Institute, Inc. *Quality Benchmarks for Executives.* Wilton, CT: Juran Institute, Inc., 1991, p. 1.

2. Milliken, R. Address on acceptance of Malcolm Baldridge National Quality Award, Washington, DC, Dec. 1989.

3. Berwick, D. M. Address to *The Healthcare Forum* Cross-QIN Meeting, San Francisco, Apr. 1993.

4. Camp, R. C. *Benchmarking: The Search for Industry Best Practices That Lead to Superior Performance.* Milwaukee, WI: ASQC [American Society for Quality Control] & Quality Resources, 1989, p. 10.

5. Camp, p. 12.

6. Hull, D. R., and Tracy, E. J. AT&T Benchmarking: Fundamental Priority. Presentation at Annual Conference of Council of Logistics Management, Anaheim, CA, 1991.

7. The SunHealth Alliance. *Benchmarking the SunHealth Way.* Charlotte, NC: The SunHealth Alliance, 1991, p. 3.

8. Catholic Health Corporation. *A Proposal to Launch Benchmarking Projects.* Omaha, NE: Catholic Health Corporation, Sept. 1992.

9. Voluntary Hospitals of America, Inc. *The Benchmarking Process.* Irving, TX: Voluntary Hospitals of America, Inc., 1992.

10. *The American Heritage Dictionary of the English Language.* New York City: Houghton Mifflin Co., 1981, p. 288.

11. Ogle, R. H. Benchmarking: A Path to Excellence. Presentation at Benchmarking: The Next Generation in Healthcare Quality, *The Healthcare Forum,* Chicago, Sept. 18, 1992.

12. Camp.

13. Spendolini, M. J. *The Benchmarking Book.* New York City: American Management Association (AMACOM), 1992.

14. Ogle.

15. Hull and Tracy.

16. Camp, p. 13.

17. Biesada, A. Benchmarking. *Financial World* 160(19):31, Sept. 17, 1991.

18. Spear, S. The emergence of learning communities. *The Systems Thinker* 3(10):1–4, 1993.

19. Spear.

20. O'Rourke, L., and Bader, B. A process for developing a board quality and performance report. *The Quality Letter* 5(2):8–14, 1993.

21. O'Rourke and Bader.

Chapter Two

Why Health Care Benchmarking?

Introduction

As described in chapter 1, benchmarking is the continual and collaborative discipline on the part of an organization of measuring, evaluating, and comparing the results of its key work processes with results of best performers. It is also a commitment to learning how to adapt best practices to the organizational culture to achieve breakthrough process improvements and ensure healthier communities. Within this definition lie the seeds of reasons why health care organizations should consider fostering competency in benchmarking.

Robert Camp of the Xerox Corporation observes that benchmarking is essentially an approach to goal setting.[1] Not only does it offer a way to determine new, attainable targets (goals); it also provides a means for identifying practices that lead to attainment of those targets.

This chapter focuses on how the practice of benchmarking fits into the current health care environment. The chapter begins by examining 10 environmental challenges with which providers are faced (from better-informed consumers to poorly defined customer populations). Next the chapter describes how benchmarking evolves once implemented and how it can help providers meet the 10 challenges discussed. Then, four industry prototypes are briefly described. The chapter closes with two benchmarking examples in health care and the dimensions in which they made breakthrough improvements.

Ten Environmental Health Care Challenges

Buffeted by waves of change from all sides, health care providers must chart a course to bring their organizations into a new era of unprecedented performance. The pace of these changes has never been quicker, their magnitude never greater.

Ten challenges in particular force providers to find new ways to "do" health care. This section briefly reviews these environmental influences so as to provide a context and establish a foundation upon which planners and administrators can increase collaboration and learning among providers. Examining these challenges promotes understanding of growing consumer demands on the nation's health care system, forcing leaders to alter how they work with others to deliver community services more cost effectively. Collectively, these challenges reflect the reasons why collaboration, learning, and breakthrough performance are critical to ensuring the well-being of health care delivery. (Note: No prioritization is intended by the numbering, which is provided for referral purposes only.)

Challenge 1: Customer Sophistication and Expectations

Today's health care consumer is better informed than ever, largely due to increased media exposure on service and care delivery. Other considerations, ranging from increased consumer awareness regarding healthier life-styles to more organizational focus on performance enhancement and quality initiatives, also contribute to customer sophistication and expectations. For example, life-style changes lead to stepped-up customer demand for a broader base of services, such as nutrition counseling, stress management, or sports medicine. Incoming health care employees from organizations that have quality improvement systems in place bring their higher expectations with them. An important dimension of patient expectations is involvement, and patients demand more information so they can make better, more informed decisions about their care and be actively engaged in treatment.

Challenge 2: Dissatisfaction in the Business Sector

Business leaders, long aware of cost shifting within health care, are dissatisfied with paying this "extra premium" for health coverage. Insurance premiums in the private sector increased by more than half as much as the total health care industry costs (1990 through 1991).[2] The financial impact of this jump is responsible for an erosion of profits that detracts from competitiveness. Consequently, pressure is on the rise for rate setting and cost controls. In a survey by the Kaiser Foundation and Commonwealth Foundation, 71 percent of respondents agreed that the government should set the rates charged by physicians and hospitals—despite evidence that price controls do nothing to contain costs.[3,4] Cost issues drive the efforts of business leaders to reshape the health care delivery system. Until costs rise at a rate less than or equal to inflation, providers can expect an increasingly adversarial relationship with purchasers.

Challenge 3: Technology–Care Schism

As technology becomes more complex and demands more user expertise and sophistication, providers are split, offering higher levels of technology but lower levels of caring compassion. The resultant situation becomes the antithesis of

Peters and Waterman's "high tech–high touch" maxim.[5] At least three potential consequences are the result of this schism. First, patients experience less satisfaction while watching costs continue to rise because of redundant technology. Second, providers create for patients the illusion of instant fixes, an expectation impossible to meet. Third, this conflict leads to an imbalance between perceived outcomes improvement relative to the increased costs. To thrive in a changing environment, providers will have to find ways to integrate technology with compassionate care.

Challenge 4: Changing Regulations and Accreditation Standards

Regulators and accrediting agencies are slowly recognizing the limitations of the traditional quality improvement inspection model imposed on health care organizations. Meanwhile, providers are faced with confusion about standard-of-care compliance. This is because the agencies, not fully versed in the new guidelines, often revert to old ones. Furthermore, agencies may change their requirements at a different pace. For example, the speed with which the JCAHO adapts their accreditation standards may exceed that of state regulating agencies.

Providers are challenged to integrate their internal strategies with "quirky" external demands until transition from old to new mandates are in sync. Advocacy efforts may accelerate uniformity of regulations, but it still may take years to reach consistency of accreditation guidelines. Until then, providers must contend with resistance and multiple demands from the numerous agencies they must deal with.

Challenge 5: Standardization in Practice Patterns and Outcomes

Studies by the Department of Community and Family Medicine at Dartmouth Medical Center and Intermountain Health Care document high rates of variation among prostectomy patients, both in terms of physician practice patterns and patient care outcomes.[6-8] As health care takes on more regional and national focus, providers are expected to reduce such variance regardless of state or region. To do this, physicians and health care facilities must implement information systems to gather and analyze patient management data, construct care protocols or care paths, and identify quality indicators. In a word, providers must begin to look beyond their own walls for standards of quality comparison and measurement.

Challenge 6: High Costs, Low Cost Performance

Since the early 1980s, U.S. health care costs have almost tripled and by the year 2000 will exceed $1.7 trillion, if current rates of increase continue.[9] Such high cost levels contribute to the decreased competition among U.S. industries. For example, in 1991 every car manufactured by the "Big Three" averaged $1,034 in health care expenses—50 percent more than the average cost of the steel used per automobile. To deal with its deficit and regain its strength as a global competitor, the United States must address runaway health care costs. Business leaders and the public alike are demanding reform in health care cost performance.

Challenge 7: Erosion of Public Trust

Growing consumer awareness of practice and outcomes variation and of rising health care costs have eroded public trust in the U.S. health care system. Although 80 percent of 2,000 respondents surveyed by the Harvard School of Public Health expressed satisfaction with the quality of care received, 56 percent support major changes to the system; 29 percent feel that total overhaul of the system is needed.[10] Faced with a public that no longer trusts the overall quality of its health care delivery system, providers must look within *and without* for a quality edge.

Challenge 8: Health Care Reform

While public sentiment supports radical change in the health care system, most consumers are skeptical that they will benefit from reform. The majority fears higher costs without concomitant higher levels of quality, or impaired quality to save costs.[11] Discussions of health care reform separate quality from costs, and within health care the debate over a presumed inverse relationship between the two continues. Other industries pursuing quality improvement do not see them as mutually exclusive. Health care reform dictated by a national policy can only bring new reimbursement methods, not revise the production process. Only those charged with stewardship of the production process can make the changes necessary to improve it.[12]

Challenge 9: Lack of Collaborative Partnership

Traditionally, with regard to medical practice and management, the relationship between hospitals and between hospitals and physicians has been competitive rather than cooperative. Despite efforts to the contrary, local health care communities continue to demonstrate antagonism more than mutuality of interests. For example, hiring functional specialists to manage upgraded or new technologies, rather than training current personnel, reinforces a hierarchical, divisive organizational structure. Studies conducted in facilities that provide patient-centered care identify two organizational needs: simplified systems and simplified service delivery support structures.[13] Such simplified delivery systems require cooperation to implement them. Patients and other customers are blind to the departmental orientation of providers, but they do see service gaps and inadequacies. Those organizations that emphasize cross-functional problem identification and process improvement are more likely to enjoy favorable customer perception of service delivery. Organizations must extend collaborative problem solving to joint efforts with other providers to reduce unnecessary duplication of services and technology, provide new services, improve community health care outcomes, and reduce overall system expense.

Challenge 10: Customer Identity, Needs, and Expectations

As explained in chapter 1, providers have not identified customers clearly. Customers include patient, physician, and payer: One uses the service; one orders it; and one pays for it—a situation unique to health care. Russ Ackoff (president of InterAct) presents a strong argument for broadening the definition of *customer* to include purchaser, consumer, employees, suppliers, shareholders, creditors, the public, and so on.[14]

The challenge is for organizations to know who their customers are, what they need and expect from providers. Assessment tools such as satisfaction surveys and community awareness campaigns help toward this end. Executive leadership teams and marketing personnel might spearhead these initiatives.

The Need for a New Approach

These 10 challenges set the stage on which health care leaders are compelled to explore solutions using new approaches. As Einstein observed, "The significant problems we have cannot be solved at the same level of thinking we were at when we created them." This premise underlies the fundamental work of leaders who must steer their facilities through the quality transformation. To create breakthrough performance and develop healthier communities, providers must endorse the discipline of collaborative benchmarking.

It is important to understand why this learning plays a significant role in helping organizations achieve world class status. As suggested in chapter 1, benchmarking is not a final destination but an evolutionary process, a concept detailed further in the next section.

The Evolution to Benchmarking

Figure 2-1 shows the evolutionary path many organizations take from initial measurement to integration of benchmarking into operations. Intervening stages in this model are comparative data and competitive analysis.

Figure 2-1. Evolution to Benchmarking

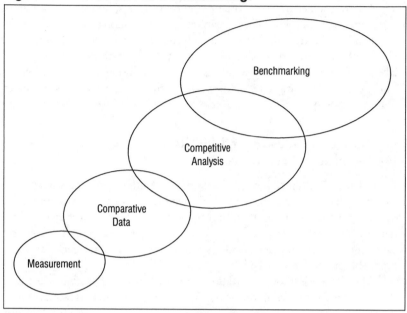

Reprinted, with permission, from the Catholic Health Corporation, Omaha, Nebraska.

Measurement

Some organizations treat the future as an extension of the past, and actual performance for one period (for example a fiscal quarter or fiscal year) provides the basis for projecting performance in the next period. With such an approach, tomorrow's performance rarely looks different from today's. Consequently, these organizations may achieve incremental improvement if any at all.

Incremental goal setting is rooted in measurement, and organizational improvement is conditioned on measurement. Measurement is not, however, sufficient in and of itself. Mostly, health care organizations use crude measures of outputs and results, which can be imprecise, retrospective, and invariably restricted to internal data.

Peter Drucker, noted management thinker, observes that most measures used in organizations are simple counts. In urging a move from counting to measuring, Drucker encourages adopting process measurement, as opposed to numbers crunching, as the means to fuller understanding of operations. Only then, he proposes, can operations be controlled and improved. As an example Drucker cites Wal-Mart's measuring the cost of an entire process, from the machine in the supplier's plant to the store's checkout counter. This measurement led to a one-third cost reduction through elimination of unnecessary paperwork and warehousing.[15]

Donald M. Berwick, MD, speaking on the progress health care organizations have made in implementing total quality management (TQM), observed that the language of measurement has begun to find usage by health care professionals. Yet, he notes, providers have yet to "domesticate measurement," to make it easy or understandable.[16] Too many organizations continue to misuse measurement, that is, using data as a stick to single out individual behavior rather than examining the production process.

Comparative Data

As organizations gain familiarity with measurement, they inevitably ask, "Are we in the ballpark?" For an answer, organizations seek comparative data. Yet, in doing so they may retain an internal focus, comparing a single period to a prior period (for example, this month to last month or this month to the same month last year). This approach may provide insight into past performance, but it has limited value for projecting long-term performance. As a snapshot, such a comparison is static and fails to provide a true moving picture of continuing performance.

As an alternative, trend analysis of internal performance measures represents an improvement over period-to-period comparisons. However, while trend analysis allows for more accurate conclusions about performance, it still lacks the external perspective.

Organizations that recognize this limitation turn their attention outside and gauge their internal performance against that of others. Because even external comparative data often appear at the local, regional, and state professional association levels and within systems or alliances, they may answer the "ballpark" question but may lack consistency and precision.

For more complete comparative data, organizations search national databases, subscription services that may include operational, clinical, and merged databases. With increased emphasis on gaining outside perspectives, some states have mandated specific comparative databases for providers. Certain precautions should be taken when relying on comparative data, as explained below.

Inaccuracies in Comparative Data

Matching "apples to oranges" ranks chief among the difficulties with comparative data. The inaccuracies that occur result from comparing measures defined differently by participating organizations. Furthermore, the operating characteristics may differ among organizations participating in a given database. For example, a foodservice department may wish to compare number of meals produced with number of labor hours worked. Some comparative databases include no means of determining whether comparisons are from straight production operations or from cook-chill or cook-freeze operations, a distinction that may influence results dramatically. Blind use of these data to compare performance and establish new targets leads to erroneous conclusions and inappropriate actions.

Indiscriminate Application of Comparative Data and Thresholds

In *Managerial Breakthrough*, Joseph M. Juran tells the following story:[17]

> During 40 historic days many kinds of animals were afloat on a certain ark. There wasn't enough to do, so someone organized study groups to make constructive use of the long hours. One of these groups got into a study of the hearts of the various animals. It turned out that there was immense variation. The big whales had huge pumps, weighing over 400 pounds; mice had tiny hearts, three thousand to the pound. This was a variation of over a million to one.
>
> Then a staff animal made a shrewd observation. "Naturally, big animals need bigger hearts. We should compare ratios—the ratio of heart weight to total body weight." They tried it out, and it worked out brilliantly. The percent of heart weight to body weight ranged from 0.1 to 0.9, a range of only 9 to 1.
>
> But the data threw consternation into the giraffe camp. Their 25-pound hearts were a thumping 0.9 percent of their body weight. The giraffe controller stated it eloquently: "Our ratio of heart weight to total body weight is twice as much as the market. We are carrying a lot of unnecessary overhead. If we could do with 15-pound hearts, we would be more in line with the market."
>
> It didn't work. Nothing but a 25-pound heart was powerful enough to pump blood to the top of an 18-foot animal.

This story points up the dangers of misapplication of comparative data. "Average" data simply cannot be taken blindly to set goals and targets but must be adapted to specific work processes and operation characteristics.

Measuring organizational performance against thresholds represents a special danger of comparative data use. Thresholds may be developed internally or mandated externally, but regardless of the source, two potentially damaging behaviors typically arise from indiscriminate application of thresholds. The first, which results from not meeting the threshold, or from being "not good enough," seeks to assign blame and sanction—neither of which fosters improvement. The second behavior results from exceeding the threshold or, ironically, from being "good enough," which can lead to the belief that no improvement is needed. Consequently, the organization complacently rests on its data laurels. Both behaviors result from measuring only outputs without examining the process that produced the outputs. In neither case does the organization get what it wants—improved performance.

Failure to Define How Results Were Achieved

Comparative databases frequently provide medians and percentiles for performance comparison purposes. These data provide points of reference, but
they do not allow determinization of the source of the better performance
so as to learn how that performance was achieved. In other words, the availability of comparative data does not equate to identifying how results were
accomplished.

Some databases circumvent this barrier by offering side-by-side reports that
allow comparison with specific organizations. The caveat here is that an organization must know which others it wants to be compared with and secure their
permission before the report can be produced. Another limitation in this
approach is that the organization compares itself to known entities, an action
with potential to preclude comparison to the superior performers. Such a report
generally compares only a few organizations that may match well in one functional area but not another; yet, comparisons are drawn for entire organizations.

Some comparative databases have taken a different approach on this issue,
requiring each department to complete an operating profile as a condition of
participation. The comparisons are then made to the departments that most
closely match the operating characteristics of the organization using the database. This change in requirement enhances the validity of data and yields more
accurate comparisons.

Other Limitations of Comparative Data

Two other limitations of comparative databases exist: departmentalization and
a median curve. Most comparative databases are structured departmentally and,
consequently, ignore the cross-functional process comparisons necessary for
improvement. A more insidious potential disadvantage lies in how data are used.
For example, in many organizations, comparative data breeds a "hit-the-median"
mentality, where the objective to reach median performance levels ignores the
potential of processes. This mentality destines an organization to mediocrity
and is inconsistent with the benchmarking mind-set.

Competitive Analysis

Organizations that experience the limitations of comparative data move to the
next evolutionary stage—competitive analysis, the examination of direct competitors. By measuring itself against market competitors, an organization can
identify its strengths and weakness. Competitive analysis also quantifies the
gaps between the subject's performance and that of its direct competitors.

Four potential drawbacks should be cautioned against with competitive
analysis. They are an industry focus, reliance on secondary data, incomplete
answers, and win–lose situations.

Industry Focus

By focusing solely on its competitors, the organization risks becoming a prisoner of its own industry. Competitive analysis focuses on what the competition has already achieved and ignores possibilities that exist outside the industry and what can be learned from other types of businesses. It also focuses the organization's energies on achieving parity with direct competitors, rather than examining best practices and looking for breakthroughs.

Reliance on Secondary Data

Because competitive analysis relies heavily on secondary information sources, it may fail to identify methods that produce the better performance of competitors. This lack of detail can lead organizations to second guess the means that produced superior performance and to take actions that are in opposition to the true practices that led to the competitors' performance. The means of improved performance are not always evident from the performance itself or from the cursory information available through competitive analysis.

Incomplete Answers

Related to secondary data is the possibility that competitive analysis can raise more questions than answers. Much of the information comes from secondary sources in the public domain, information that may be inconsistent, incomplete, and antiquated. In addition, analysts studying the organization's competitors may bring preconceived notions into the process, a mind-set that may lead them to obtain data that support the prevailing view rather than reflect the true situation. Finally, competitor analysis ultimately can end in a mountain of data but little useful information.

Win–Lose Situations

The U.S. business arena is inherently competitive, operating on an either–or ("win–lose") presumption in the market. This presumption of antagonism over collaboration contributes to the challenges facing the health care environment. Such an attitude impedes a customer focus and, ultimately, improved health care available to the community.

Although it is not the most effective way for organizations to identify goals and achieve breakthrough improvements, competitive analysis is a useful tool in certain situations. Like other methodologies, it must be selected and applied appropriately. Wallecke explores its proper role in improving business performance in his article "A Backstage View of World-Class Performers."[18]

Benchmarking

The evolutionary path from measurement to comparative data to competitive analysis culminates with benchmarking. However, the progression to and discipline of benchmarking goes further, to determine not only best performance but the practices that create that best performance.

Organizations that measure, compare data, and analyze competitors most often relegate these practices to staff functions. Companies that use benchmarking successfully make it the role of line functions and the operators within the processes being studied. This involvement invests workers in the improvement sought, the practices discovered, and the actions instituted. Benchmarking is not a spectator sport; it requires the active participation of those involved in the area under investigation. As always, it promotes looking to other industries and disciplines for best practices—or, to borrow a phrase from Michael Spendolini's *The Benchmarking Book,* "thinking outside the box."[19]

Reasons for Benchmarking in Health Care

Chapter 1 described factors in the health care operating environment that demand change in the delivery of health care services. To make these changes, improvement of breakthrough proportion is required. This fact represents the overarching reason to conduct benchmarking studies. This and other reasons are discussed in the following sections.

Breakthrough Performance

Benchmarking is uniquely qualified to help organizations identify best practices that lead to breakthrough performance improvements. Such improvements require second-order change over first-order change.

First-order change is a term used by psychotherapist Paul Watzlawick to describe changes made to return to homeostasis.[20] In the context of quality improvement, these incremental improvements of existing processes achieve stability and reduce variation. First-order changes have become the primary thrust of many organizational quality initiatives. Unfortunately, these initiatives fail to question the entire process, and it is such questioning that leads to second-order changes.

Second-order change moves organizations to higher levels of performance, not just incrementally but in orders of magnitude. If first-order changes are those made *within* the system, then second-order changes are those made *to* the system.

An example that clarifies the distinction is a hospital's examination of its admitting process. Assume that the current process takes 40 minutes to register inpatients and escort them to their rooms. Improving efficiency within the system so that the process takes only 20 minutes exemplifies first-order change, with patients continuing to experience the same process. In a different scenario, assume that the patient is met at the door and escorted directly to the room without having to go to an admitting department. Intake information is gathered one time only, at the bedside, and only one patient signature is required. Assume further that all these activities occur within 10 minutes. This exemplifies second-order change: the system has been changed dramatically, as has the experience—both for provider and recipient.

Benchmarking uncovers practices that lead to second-order change. That means substantial modification of existing processes and the push for organizations to achieve breakthrough levels of performance.

Goal and Target Credibility

As mentioned at the beginning of this chapter, benchmarking is fundamentally a planning process, an alternative way to set goals and targets. Tightly connected to the best-in-class outcomes in the external environment, benchmarking results in goals and targets based in the reality of superior performance. These goals and targets stem from repeated analytic evaluation against best practices and are consistent with customer requirements. Therefore, they have more credibility with managers and staff.

Customer Focus

The rigor of benchmarking helps organizations better define customer requirements in specific terms. As a result, the organization complements its internal focus with outside perspectives. This increased sensitivity to changes in the external environment better positions the organization for anticipating and responding to community needs.

Improved Decision Making

Enhanced knowledge about customer and community needs leads to better decision making by organizational leaders. Thus, the organization can more wisely allocate limited resources so as to better respond to customer needs. Because its knowledge of these demands is rooted in fact and not speculation, the organization gains confidence in its decision-making abilities.

Process Focus

Benchmarking reinforces a focus on process while keeping the desired outcomes firmly in mind. By first comparing the results and then the processes that produce these results, benchmarking identifies best practices. Adaptation of best practices into operations makes breakthrough improvement possible. Benchmarking, then, focuses on the processes and practices that produce superior performance.

Identification of Performance Measures

Identifying performance measures that accurately address customer demands results in more objective measures of performance at all levels. Measures based on real practices elsewhere have more credibility than those set using comparative data or internal historical practice. Determined by participants and witnessed in action in benchmarking partners' operations, these performance measures become more readily adoptable. Benchmarking, then, helps convince planners and administrators of the operational accuracy of these measures.

Innovation and Creativity

Some critics blast benchmarking as merely a form of emulation that stifles innovation. This criticism plays out peculiarly in health care organizations, specifically with the issue of clinical pathways. Assailed as "cookbook medicine," pathways (or patient care protocols) may be unacceptable to clinicians protective of their autonomy. Faced with the superior results achieved through pathways, however, these same clinicians are more likely to embrace them. Furthermore, pathways provide a springboard to service delivery enhancements, incorporating innovations created by practicing clinicians.

When a benchmarking team identifies what is possible and understands the reasons for the performance gap, creativity is enhanced. Organizations experienced with benchmarking attest to its ability to stir creativity by eliminating self-imposed barriers, which in turn reinforces a culture that values continuous improvement. A sense of urgency is created by identifying how others perform and seeing the gap between an organization's performance and that of superior organizations. Rather than demotivating benchmarking proponents, this knowledge pushes participants to close the gap.

Cooperation

Again, benchmarking encourages cooperation among organizations. As associates from different organizations participate on benchmarking projects, collaborative relationships emerge to expand the resource networks of participants, which in turn aids future problem solving and improvement efforts. More important, they build bridges between organizations and represent avenues for further collaboration to achieve learning and enhance knowledge.

Prototypes for Benchmarking Success

Studying and adapting the business practices of other companies is a strategy that organizations have been doing, formally and informally, for years. Benchmarking takes this concept and creates a framework for increasing its success potential. The following models—Ford, Xerox Corporation, and Chrysler—demonstrate how firmly entrenched in industrial development the practice is.

Henry Ford

Henry Ford reportedly came upon the idea for developing his automobile assembly line after visiting a slaughterhouse. The cattle were hung on a J-hook suspended from a track at one end of the slaughterhouse, and as the track wound its way around the slaughterhouse floor, butchers at workstations removed portions of meat until the carcass was disassembled. Ford envisioned this process in reverse and came up with the plan for his automobile assembly operation.

Ford also borrowed ideas from other successful firms of his day. In doing so, he identified an important benchmarking principle: It is crucial to examine how the best practice will fit within a current operation system. Simply installing an assembly line, however, did not yield the results Ford sought; in fact, doing so created other problems. Assembling a car in this manner required that parts be brought to the workstations in a timely and accurate fashion. Having too few parts or the wrong parts stopped the line; conversely, too many parts crowded the workstations. To resolve the inventory management problem, Ford contacted a leader in inventory control at the time – Sears Roebuck – and adapted techniques learned into his automobile assembly operation.

Xerox Corporation

With the introduction of xerography, Xerox was in the enviable position of having dominated world markets. Given marketplace fragility, however, Xerox soon found its position had eroded, as shown in figure 2-2, which compares selected dimensions of Xerox's performance for 1975 and 1981. Virtually every area at the company showed decline over this six-year period. In a fiercely competitive industry, Xerox faced the challenge of fundamentally changing the way it conducted business. The significant event was finding Japanese products in the United States that sold for less than it cost Xerox to make them.

In 1981, Xerox managers visited Japan to better understand the competition. Figure 2-3 compares Xerox and Japanese competitors in specific areas identified during that visit. The most important lesson learned was the need for the American company to go behind the numbers in defining the different

Figure 2-2. The Xerox Experience

	1975	1981
Market share	85%	35%
Profitability	Above average	Below average
Growth rate	15%+	Marginal
Product line	State of the art	Obsolete
Stock price	30× earnings	"The pits"
Recommendation	Buy	Sell
Competition	Few, poor quality	Fierce

Adapted, with permission, from *Benchmarking: The Success Analysis Tool,* published by The James Group, Scottsdale, Arizona, copyright 1991.

levels of performance. This action, *studying the processes that produced the results,* made the effort more than just another competitive analysis.

Between 1981 and 1987, Xerox worked to implement benchmarking into its corporate operations. Beginning with benchmarking of costs industrywide, the discipline spread quickly across all operations areas. Yet, even with the success that followed, it took Xerox more than four years to fully institutionalize the practice. The performance improvements that came as a result of benchmarking studies were communicated widely, both within and outside the corporation. Company officials credit benchmarking as the primary reason for Xerox's resurgence.

Figure 2-4 shows the company's 1989 performance for the same dimensions reported for 1975 and 1981 (see figure 2-2, p. 30). Xerox continues to prosper in an industry where competition remains intense, largely due to the company's ability to learn from others collaboratively. In addition to improving

Figure 2-3. Xerox–Japan Comparison (1981)

Characteristic	Japan	Xerox
Product design	Concurrent	Sequential
Part flexibility	Interchangeable	Model dependent
Parts involved	"X"	"1.8X"
Suppliers	200	4,000+
Cost to make	"Y"	"2Y"
Staffing: direct to nondirect	7 to 1	2 to 1

Adapted, with permission, from *Benchmarking: The Success Analysis Tool,* published by The James Group, Scottsdale, Arizona, copyright 1991.

Figure 2-4. Xerox Breakthroughs (1989)

	1989
Market share	46%
Profitability	Above average
Growth rate	Faster than market
Product line	Focused
Stock price	Above average
Recommendation	Buy
Competition	46 worldwide

Adapted, with permission, from *Benchmarking: The Success Analysis Tool,* published by The James Group, Scottsdale, Arizona, copyright 1991.

its own performance, Xerox serves as an example, to all companies in all indus-tries, of the power that collaborative learning through a structured benchmarking discipline can bring.

Chrysler

A less-publicized but equally successful benchmarking application occurred at the Chrysler Corporation. "Chrysler's drive back to the top has been a long and winding road,"[21] reads the lead in an article describing Chrysler's success. A significant contributor to that success was a two-year benchmarking study with Honda Motor Company. Chrysler chose Honda because of similarities in organizational size and in the limited product line each company offers. From that benchmarking study, Chrysler learned lessons about lean production, lean management, and new approaches to product development and then utilized these approaches in developing its new automobile line.

By developing a network of suppliers, Chrysler accessed their talents to identify innovations and reduce costs. Company leaders relied on this network to offset product development costs. Another lesson learned dealt with struc-ture. Chrysler replaced its traditional functional hierarchy with cross-disciplinary teams empowered to challenge traditional approaches to product component development. Team efforts produced astounding results, one of which was at the component level, where an indicator readout system was created with all the advantages of electronic systems – but at a cost less than existing mechani-cal ones.

Results at the production level are even more impressive. Teams designed and engineered the product line for $1.7 billion, less than one third the cost of previous efforts. The program at its peak involved 744 staff, less than half the budgeted 1,500 positions. The time from concept approval to production, typically five years, was reduced to just 39 months. Most important, the effort produced an automobile that is innovative, cost-effective, and in high demand.

The product development system that the teams identified, adapted, and implemented represents the best in the U.S. automobile industry. That system positioned Chrysler to introduce more innovative products at a faster pace than competing manufacturers. For example, it allowed Chrysler to introduce a cab-forward sub-compact model that may be the first profitable U.S.-produced small car in years.

Other, broader benchmarking successes are observable throughout indus-try. Some are fairly matter of fact; others may be apocryphal. For example, Xerox studied distribution from L.L. Bean; Motorola gained insight into delivery processes from Domino's Pizza; and Southwest Airlines, trying to speed air-plane turnaround time, learned from pit crews at the Indianapolis 500 Race-way. Whether true or the stuff of benchmarking lore, the point remains that opportunities to learn abound for those who are open to seeing them.

Two Health Care Benchmarking Pioneers

A few health care benchmarking pioneers are opening doors for others to follow. The two cases that follow exemplify early work conducted in the field.

Elective Acute Care Inpatient Admitting Process

In January 1992, The Healthcare Forum (THF) and the American Productivity and Quality Center's (APQC) International Benchmarking Clearinghouse collaborated to conduct a benchmarking study of the elective acute care inpatient admitting process.[22] The study involved members of THF's Quality Improvement Networks (QINs).

This benchmarking project was organized into two phases. In the first phase, practice dimensions from 28 participants were identified and catalogued. This data-gathering process led to identifying the best practices among the group. Findings included identification of critical success factors; process enablers and inhibitors; and recommended measures for effectiveness, efficiency, and economy.

The second phase involved identifying cross-industry models of effectiveness that could be translated for application in health care. Industries studied included hotels, airlines, car rental companies, and insurance companies. This study resulted in identifying those lessons learned from non–health care settings that had similar work processes that health care providers could use to accelerate performance of the inpatient elective acute care admitting process to breakthrough levels.

Two organizations have demonstrated improved operations as a direct result of participation in the benchmarking project. St. Mary's Hospital Medical Center (Madison, Wisconsin) now preadmits 97 percent of its patients, compared with 55 percent previously. Time required to admit patients is now less than a minute and a half, a reduction of 85 percent.[23] St. Joseph's Medical Center (Stockton, California) reports that patients interact with one fewer staff member due to cross training, reduced overtime due to fewer chart inspections, and reduced bad debts.[24]

Emergency Services

The SunHealth Alliance (Charlotte, North Carolina) comprises 240 hospitals and other health care organizations located primarily in the southeastern United States. Fifteen members of the alliance joined forces to conduct two benchmarking studies where participants learned the benefits of group benchmarking. The chief executive officers of the participating facilities selected topics of importance to the organizations, one of which was emergency services.

In the emergency services study the group identified keys to improved performance, including the following:

- Strong triage systems to speed identification of patient needs and placement for treatment. This system requires staff with diverse skills to work together to accomplish this goal.
- Standardized nursing protocols to allow nurses to initiate orders for selected diagnostic tests before the physician sees the patient. This provides more complete information for the physician and reduces patient waiting time.
- Ancillary services located near the emergency department to speed service delivery.
- Patient tracking systems that permit staff to know where the patient is at all times.

The lessons learned from this study allowed redesign of emergency systems to increase patient satisfaction and improve care.[25,26]

Summary

The future of health care includes managed competition and integrated delivery networks. It also includes more astute and demanding customers and purchasers. For organizations to prosper under these evolving conditions they must meet and exceed the requirements and expectations (better outcomes, reduced costs, improved value, and so on) of their customers.

In addition, health care organizations must develop characteristics that ensure their viability in the marketplace. For example, they must become more flexible to accommodate increasingly diverse service demands from customers and more responsive to withstand market shifts. To develop these and other abilities, organizations must learn from their customers and competitors in addition to learning from themselves. Collaborative learning and collaborative networks will help identify opportunities, solve problems, and provide services to improve community well-being. The vehicle of choice toward these goals is collaborative benchmarking.

Putting These Ideas to Work

Objective

Identify the driving forces that motivate your organization to initiate benchmarking and the restraining forces that could inhibit the process.

This activity will help clarify the reasons why an organization chooses to proceed. It will also help identify the barriers to success that must be overcome.

Approach

Using force-field analysis, state the desired action, for example, initiate benchmarking studies. Brainstorm the driving forces, those that propel the stated action toward becoming a reality. Repeat the brainstorming process, this time focusing on the restraining forces, those obstacles that block forward movement.

Discuss the driving forces to determine their relative impact. Multivoting, forced ranking, or open discussion can be helpful in this activity. Repeat this discussion activity with the restraining forces.

The resulting list of driving forces are those issues, ranked by priority, that encourage proceeding with benchmarking. These represent leverage points for selling the discipline to the various constituencies of the organization. The resulting list of restraining forces are those issues, also ranked by priority, that discourage proceeding with benchmarking. These represent the barriers the organization must overcome if it is to succeed in this effort.

Both lists represent valuable insights into communications and cultural change issues that must be addressed. Figure 2-5 presents a format to facilitate this discussion and display the force field-analysis graphically.

For purposes of this and subsequent work activities, the authors assume that readers have a working familiarity with the basic tools of quality improvement. The notes at the end of the chapter contain additional references on the tools.[27]

Figure 2-5. Force-Field Analysis

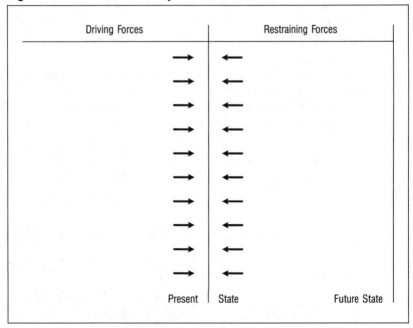

Reprinted, with permission, from the Catholic Health Corporation, Omaha, Nebraska.

References and Notes

1. Camp, R. C. *Benchmarking: The Search for Industry Best Practices That Lead to Superior Performance.* Milwaukee, WI: ASQC & Quality Resources, 1989. p 28.

2. Congressional Budget Office. *Economic Implications of Rising Health Care Costs.* Washington, DC: Government Publishing Office, Oct. 1992.

3. Kaiser Foundation and Commonwealth Foundation. Health Insurance Survey–1992. Oakland, CA: Kaiser Foundation and Commonwealth Foundation, 1992.

4. Grayson, C. J. Experience talks: shun price controls. . . . *Wall Street Journal*, March 29, 1993, p. B4.

5. Peters, T. J., and Waterman, R. H., Jr. *In Search of Excellence.* New York City: Harper & Row, Publishers, 1982.

6. Wennberg, J. E., Mulley, A. G., and others. An assessment of prostatectomy for benign urinary tract obstruction: Geographic variations and the evaluation of medical care outcomes. *JAMA* 259(20):3027–30, May 27, 1988.

7. Lu-Yao, G. L., McLerran, D., Wasson, J., and Wennberg, J. E., for the Prostate Patient Outcomes Research Team. An assessment of radical prostatectomy: time trends, geographic variation, and outcomes. *JAMA* 269(20):2633–36, 1993.

8. James, B. C. *Quality Management for Health Care Delivery.* Chicago: The Hospital Research and Educational Trust, 1984, pp. 21–22.

9. Data from the Congressional Budget Office, Washington, DC, 1992.

10. Unpublished survey of 2,000 Americans conducted by the Harvard School of Public Health, funded by the Robert Wood Johnson Foundation, Mar. 18–25, 1993.

11. Unpublished Harvard survey.

12. Comments made by Donald M. Berwick, MD, president and chief executive officer of the Institute for Healthcare Improvement, during a presentation entitled, "Quality Convictions: Beyond the Beginning" at the meeting Quality Improvement Network of The Healthcare Forum, San Francisco, CA, Apr. 21, 1993.

13. Lathrop, J. P. The patient-focused hospital. *Healthcare Forum Journal* 34(4):17–21, July–Aug. 1991.

14. Ackoff, R. L. Beyond total quality management. *The Journal for Quality and Participation* 16(2):66–78, Mar. 1993.

15. Drucker, P. F. We need to measure, not count. *Wall Street Journal*, Apr. 13, 1993, p. B4.

16. Comments made by Donald M. Berwick, MD.

17. Juran, J. M. *Managerial Breakthrough.* McGraw-Hill Book Company, 1964, pp. 243–44.

18. Walleck, S. A. A Backstage View of World-Class Performers. The McKinsey Quarterly Reprint Series, McKinsey & Company, 1991.

19. Spendolini, M. J. *The Benchmarking Book.* New York City: AMACOM, 1992, p. 23.

20. Watzlawick, P., Wealdand, J. H., and Fisch, R. *Change: Principles of Problem Formation and Problem Resolution.* New York City: Norton, 1974.

21. Eisenstein, P. A. The driving force behind Chrysler's turnaround. *HEMISPHERE*, June 1993, pp. 29–31.

22. The Healthcare Forum and the American Productivity and Quality Center: Benchmarking for Healthcare Improvement–The Elective Acute Care Inpatient Admitting Process. The Healthcare Forum, San Francisco, CA, 1992.

23. Somers, M. Acting on Results: Admitting Process Breakthroughs, presentation given at Benchmarking: The Next Generation in Healthcare Quality Improvement, Chicago, Aug. 17–20, 1993.

24. Mitchell, L. Acting on Results: Admitting Process Breakthroughs, presentation given at Benchmarking: The Next Generation in Healthcare Improvement, Chicago, Aug. 17–20, 1993.

25. O'Rourke, L. M. Healthcare organizations adapt benchmarking techniques from industry to make quality gains. *The Quality Letter*, Sept. 1992, pp. 2–10.

26. Patrick, M. S. Benchmarking–Targeting "Best Practices." *The Healthcare Forum Journal* 35(4):71–72, July–Aug. 1992.

27. For explanations and examples of the quality improvement tools, many fine references exist. Among those are: Leebov, W., and Ersoz, C. J. *The Health Care Manager's Guide to Continuous Quality Improvement.* Chicago: American Hospital Publishing, 1991. Mizuno, S., ed. *Management for Quality Improvement.* Cambridge, MA: Productivity Press, 1988. Plsek, P. E., and Onnias, A. *Quality Improvement Tools.* Wilton, CT: Juran Institute, 1989. Productivity-Quality Systems and QIP. *Total Quality Transformation Improvement Tools.* Miamisburg, OH: Productivity-Quality Systems, 1992.

Part Two

The Collaborative Benchmarking Model

Chapter Three

Overview of the Collaborative Benchmarking Model

Introduction

Chapters 1 and 2 described the rationale for benchmarking in health care, the potential of a collaborative approach, and the conditions for success. This brief chapter is an overview of the collaborative benchmarking model as it pertains to health care. Each of the four phases summarized here will be discussed in chapters 4–7.

The Model

Collaborative benchmarking occurs in four phases, as shown in figure 3-1. Phase 1 is selection of the benchmarking topic; phase 2 is establishment of the collaborative; phase 3 is the internal benchmarking study; and phase 4 is the external study, either within the industry or across industries. Phases 3 and 4 of the model are built on Shewhart's PDSA cycle (described below).

Phase 1: Select the Benchmarking Topic

The selection of a study topic or focus initiates the benchmarking process (detailed in chapter 4). In most cases, the topic for a project is chosen by an organization (the project sponsor) before the collaborative is formed.

Phase 2: Establish the Collaborative

The sponsor solicits interest in the selected topic on the part of potential organizational participants. Forming the collaborative among health care organizations that have a common interest in the topic helps ensure resources and support for the study. This phase is detailed in chapter 5.

Phase 3: Conduct an Internal Study

Conducting a project study within the collaborative has a dual purpose: to foster understanding on the part of each participant organization of the process

Figure 3-1. Collaborative Benchmarking Model

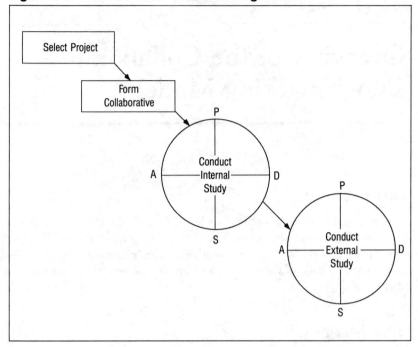

being studied and to identify best practices within the collaborative (the subjects of chapter 6). Any best practices disclosed by the internal study are adapted and implemented, then evaluated to determine whether the desired performance was achieved. If not, the collaborative generally proceeds with an external study.

Phase 4: Conduct an External Study

In examining approaches of partners outside the collaborative, participants seek to determine best practices that members of the collaborative will adapt to achieve breakthrough results. External partners may be other health care organizations or non-health care entities. This final phase of the model is covered in chapter 7.

The process used in both the internal and external study phases of collaborative benchmarking is an adaptation of the Shewhart cycle—Plan-Do-Study-Act. The PDSA cycle (the scientific method) is used not only to guide both iterations of the study, it is applied at key points within the study, such as implementing best practices. The Shewhart cycle was selected for its proven effectiveness as an improvement methodology both within and outside health care. Of equal importance, using the PDSA cycle has the advantage of applying a model and language already familiar to many health care managers and most quality professionals. Hopefully this strategy will build on existing experience, facilitate conversation about benchmarking in health care, and make learning and applying the approach more efficient.

Key Participants and Their Responsibilities

Generally speaking, various activities of the benchmarking process are "owned" by key groups involved in the project. For example:

- *Sponsoring organization:* The organization that identifies the study topic and initiates formation of the collaborative
- *Collaborative:* Key decision makers who represent the participating organizations
- *Guidance team:* In a large collaborative (more than 15 participants), a steering committee that plans and directs the project; in a smaller one, the key decision makers may fulfill this role
- *Quality council:* The senior management team of each participating organization that sets decision-making criteria
- *Benchmarking team:* The study team in each organization
- *Site visit team:* The study team representing the collaborative in the external study and site visit

Figure 3-2 shows where primary ownership lies with respect to steps in the collaborative benchmarking approach.

A Step-by-Step Guide through Each Phase

Figures 3-3 through 3-6 (pp. 45–50) summarize at-a-glance the steps, or activities, that comprise each phase of the model. In addition, the figures spell out what each step involves, who is responsible for carrying out the step, and what tools or strategies might be used to fulfill that step.

Putting These Ideas to Work

Objective

Determine the areas in which you or key decision makers in your organization could use further learning to facilitate your success with benchmarking.

Approach

1. Working alone or together, use this chapter as a "knowledge checklist" to identify the phases and/or steps of collaborative benchmarking you need to learn about before proceeding as project participants.

Figure 3-2. "Ownership" of Key Participants in a Collaborative Benchmarking Model

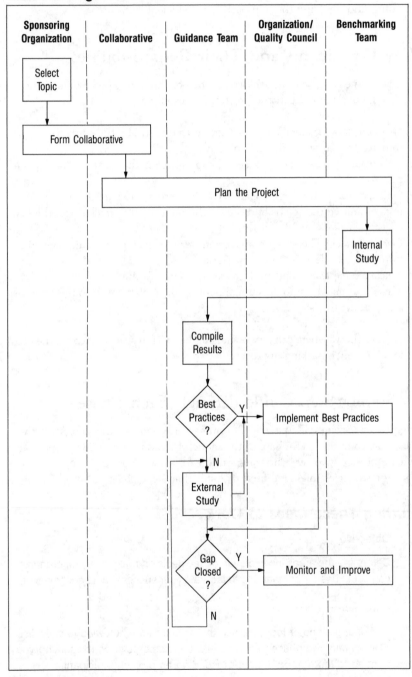

2. Assign the appropriate chapter(s) or sections of a chapter to be read and presented by members of your council or decision-making group.
3. Present the key ideas of the assigned reading for discussion.
4. Agree on actions to be taken to further your learning about methods or tools identified in the readings.

Figure 3-3. Phase 1: Project Selection

Select the Benchmarking Project (Chapter 4)			
Step	**Responsibility**	**Description**	**Tool/Strategy**
• Develop decision criteria	SO	Develop criteria to guide selection of project & reduce list of potential projects	Brainstorming Consensus
• Generate list of potential study topics	SO	Identify potential benchmarking projects from key work processes, strategic issues, critical outcomes	Brainstorming Pareto analysis
• Apply decision criteria	SO	Shorten candidate list	Rank order Decision matrix
• Agree on project focus	SO	Senior managers in sponsoring organization agree on project	Consensus

Key: SO = Sponsoring organization   PO = Participating organization
           BC = Benchmarking collaborative   BT = Benchmarking team
           GT = Guidance team   SVT = Site visit team

Figure 3-4. Phase 2: Formation of Collaborative

Establish the Benchmarking Collaborative (Chapter 5)			
Step	Responsibility	Description	Tool/Strategy
• Determine level of interest in forming a collaborative	SO	Test support for the collaborative in the sponsoring organization	Dialogue
• Identify potential participant organizations	SO	Identify potential members of collaborative	Inquiry in networks, system or alliance Brainstorming
• Identify key decision makers	SO	Identify managers who can commit to participation	Check management rosters
• Explore and generate interest in project and collaborative	SO	Explore interest of key decision makers in joining collaborative	Presentation Inquiry
• Confirm participants	SO	Confirm collaborative membership; if insufficient interest, continue to explore	Consensus Inquiry
• Identify stakeholders	BC	Identify individual & group stakeholders in project; plan for inclusion	Brainstorming Check organizational rosters
• Create collaborative project charter	BC	Develop mission, expected results, participation requirements, key dates; identify process boundaries and guidance team	Planning Gantt chart
• Adopt a benchmarking ethics code	BC	The collaborative commits itself to operate by a standard set of principles for benchmarking	Benchmarking code of conduct
• Select the guidance team	BC	Determine size of guidance team and select collaborative representatives to serve as members	Dialogue Consensus

Key: SO = Sponsoring organization   PO = Participating organization
       BC = Benchmarking collaborative   BT = Benchmarking team
       GT = Guidance team   SVT = Site visit team

Figure 3-5. Phase 3: Internal Study

Conduct the Benchmarking Study—Internal (Chapter 6)			
Plan			
Step	**Responsibility**	**Description**	**Tool/Strategy**
• Select process owner	PO	Identify logical owner of process	High-level flowchart
• Select benchmarking team	PO	Identify those with knowledge of the process	High-level flowchart
• Develop work plan	PO	Incorporate project mission, key performance indicators, project road map, budget	Use project charter Gantt chart/project planning
• Provide resources	PO	Identify resource requirements of team—time, travel, consultant, software, etc.	Budgeting/project planning
• Develop study charter	PO	Prepare summary document of mission, road map, budget, etc.	Charter framework
• Identify stakeholders	PO, BT	Identify individual & group stakeholders in project; plan for inclusion	Brainstorming Check organizational rosters
• Communicate with stakeholders	PO, BT	Inform organization of project, team and study plans	Management meetings Newsletters
• Prepare the team	GT, PO	Provide training in benchmarking methods and tools	Orientation Just-in-time teaching Benchmarking model Process analysis tools Team development Decision tools
Do			
• Describe current process	BT	Document operation of current work process	High-level flowchart Detail flowchart
• Identify key customers	BT	Identify those who depend on the outputs of the process	High-level and detail flowcharts
• Identify key output characteristics (KOCs)	BT	Document and prioritize requirements and determine key measures of performance	Focus groups, surveys, interviews Affinity diagram Interrelationship digraph Prioritization matrixes

(Continued on next page)

Figure 3-5.   (Continued)

Do *(Continued)*			
Step	**Responsibility**	**Description**	**Tool/Strategy**
• Identify process variables	BT	Identify variables which affect process performance	Cause-effect diagram Tree diagram
• Plan data collection	BT	Determine information needed and plan for collecting data	Data collection planning questions Data sheet Checksheet
• Test data collection plan	BT	Evaluate data collection plan; revise as necessary	P-D-S-A
• Collect data	BT	Implement data collection plan	Data collection plan and component tools
Study			
• Analyze performance data	BT	Ensure process stability; identify key process variables and process enablers	Run chart Control chart Pareto analysis Histogram Scatter diagram
• Compile results	BT/GT	Gather results of organizational studies	Summary data display Charts and graphs Spider diagram
• Compare performance	GT	Analyze performance of collaborative participants to determine if best practices are present; identify performance gap	Comparative analysis of results Gap analysis—"Z" chart
Act			
• Implement best practices, if any	BT, PO	Benchmarking teams implement any best practices found within the collaborative	Planning Force-field analysis Redesign 7 management planning tools P-D-S-A
• Monitor performance	PO	Plan to hold performance gains	Data collection Data analysis
• Continue to improve	PO	Plan for continuing improvement of performance	P-D-S-A

Key: SO = Sponsoring organization   PO = Participating organization
       BC = Benchmarking collaborative   BT = Benchmarking team
       GT = Guidance team   SVT = Site visit team

Figure 3-6. Phase 4: External Study

Conduct the Benchmarking Study—External (Chapter 7)			
Plan			
Step	**Responsibility**	**Description**	**Tool/Strategy**
• Develop work plan	GT	Develop work plan as in internal cycle of study	Use project charter Gantt chart/project planning
• Clarify questions	GT	Determine questions to answer to ensure breakthrough performance	Data on performance gaps Customer knowledge Process knowledge Prioritization/decision matrixes Consensus
• Determine study type	GT, BC	Determine whether to benchmark within the industry or outside	Mission/project charter Gap analysis Process knowledge Consensus
• Conduct research to identify potential partners	GT	Search primary and secondary sources to identify possible partners which meet criteria	Networking Surveys/interviews/focus groups Library/data base research Data matrix
• Screen and select potential partners	GT, BC	Screening criteria are used to identify a list of six–eight prospective partners	Selection criteria Decision matrix Consensus
• Develop questionnaires and interview guides	GT	Questionnaires and interview guides are developed to focus surveys, telephone interviews, and site visits	Surveys Focus groups Fax/computer communication Site visits
• Request participation	GT	The participation of prospective partners is formally solicited	Request letter Benchmarking questions
• Plan site visits	GT, SVT	The site visit is carefully planned to optimize the visit	Scheduling matrix Meeting agenda Role assignments Confirming letter Information packet
Do			
• Conduct site visit(s)	SVT	The site visit is conducted, following the plan developed earlier	Meeting agenda Logistics management Respect for culture Common language Management of roles Time management Benchmarking code of conduct

(Continued on next page)

Figure 3-6. (Continued)

		Do *(Continued)*	
Step	**Responsibility**	**Description**	**Tool/Strategy**
• Site visit follow-up	SVT, BC	Site visit team thanks partner, conducts a debriefing session, documents the visit, and reports to the collaborative	Common debriefing and site visit report formats Conference call, video teleconference, E-mail
		Study	
• Compile results	SVT, GT	Gather results of organizational studies	Summary data display Charts and graphs Spider diagram
• Compare performance; identify best practices	GT	Analyze performance of partners to identify best practices and process enablers; identify performance gap	Comparative analysis of results Gap analysis—"Z" chart
• Communicate best practices	GT, BC	Best practices and enablers are communicated to collaborative members	Benchmarking study summary Report sessions
		Act	
• Implement best practices	BT, PO	Benchmarking teams implement best practices found among partners; stakeholders are informed of study results and plans for improvement	Planning Force-field analysis Redesign 7 management planning tools P–D–S–A
• Monitor performance	PO	Plan to hold performance gains	Data collection Data analysis
• Continue to improve	PO, GT	Plan for continuing improvement of performance; a final project report is prepared	P–D–S–A
• Next steps	BC	The collaborative decides whether to conclude or to continue	"Lessons learned" dialogue Consensus Repeat of benchmarking process Concluding ritual

Key: SO = Sponsoring organization   PO = Participating organization
      BC = Benchmarking collaborative   BT = Benchmarking team
      GT = Guidance team   SVT = Site visit team

Bibliography

AT&T. *Benchmarking: Focus on World-Class Practices.* Indianapolis, IN: AT&T Quality Steering Committee, 1992.

Benchmarking the Best. Houston, TX: American Productivity & Quality Center, International Benchmarking Clearinghouse, 1993.

Camp, R. C. *Benchmarking: The Search for Industry Best Practices That Lead to Superior Performance.* Milwaukee, WI: ASQC & Quality Resources, 1989.

GOAL/QPC. *Memory Jogger.* Methuen, MA: GOAL/QPC, 1988.

GOAL/QPC. *The Memory Jogger Plus.* Methuen, MA: GOAL/QPC, 1989.

Leebov, W., and Ersoz, C. J., eds. *The Health Care Manager's Guide to Continuous Quality Improvement.* Chicago: American Hospital Publishing, 1991.

Spendolini, M. *The Benchmarking Book.* New York City: AMACOM, 1992.

Phase 1: Select the Project

Introduction

"What you benchmark should be of strategic importance; a competitive area; a critical success factor; a problem area; or significant in terms of quality, cost, or cycle time."[1] This quote provides insight into what should be benchmarked and why. The purpose of benchmarking is to attain superior performance in areas important to the customer. Health care organizations need to focus their benchmarking efforts in a way that accomplishes this purpose. Joseph M. Juran, in discussing the "vital few and trivial many," emphasizes the importance of identifying and acting on the issues critical to organizational success.[2] Organizations must follow this counsel and concentrate their benchmarking efforts on the "vital few" important issues.

Time limitations for improvement efforts, the direct costs incurred with benchmarking studies, and the large number of issues that compete for managerial attention are three key reasons to select the right project—the one that delivers breakthrough improvements in areas critical to meeting customer needs. This chapter provides a step-by-step guide through phase 1—how an organization can identify the projects that best fit its needs.

The steps delineated for phase 1 comprise an approach that senior leaders can follow to ensure that the project selected improves organizational performance significantly. (See figure 4-1.) Although this approach is shown in the context of the benchmarking collaborative, it also applies to individual organizations that wish to initiate benchmarking projects.

First, senior leaders develop a framework for decision making, in effect, to "decide how they are going to decide." Decision criteria delineates which conditions the group wants the benchmarking project to meet before allotting the resources necessary to conduct the project. Without identifying and weighting these criteria, candidates for study topics cannot be determined accurately.

Second, the leaders generate a list of potential projects (study topics) from several sources, a process discussed in a later section. The third step involves applying the weighted decision criteria to the list of candidate topics. This step eliminates those projects that absolutely do not meet the conditions, thus

Figure 4-1.   Select the Benchmarking Project

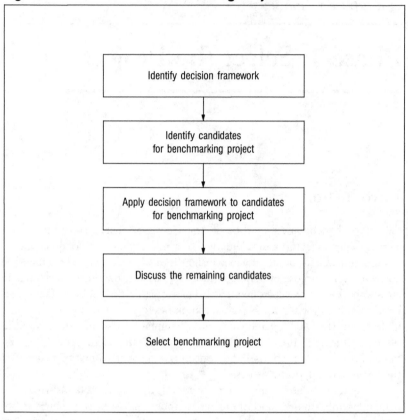

reducing the number of alternatives and focusing group discussion on remaining ones. From this remainder list the senior leaders reach agreement on the project (or projects) for benchmarking. Following this framework ensures group consensus for the project.

Step 1: Identify and Weight Decision Criteria

Health care organizations are faced with a number of issues that can benefit from breakthrough improvements. Quality, cost, and customer satisfaction are only three possible areas. To maximize the appropriate use of resources and the return on benchmarking efforts, the senior management team must select and rate projects wisely.

To do so they first must determine selection criteria, those conditions that projects must meet (independent of the specific criteria for individual projects). Judicious selection avoids "cutting the bottom to fit the britches," that is, fitting decisions around preconceived conditions. The purpose of these conditions is to cull the list of potential benchmarking candidates so that decision makers reach more focused consensus on final project selection.

Concurrent with the selection process, the team must develop weights for rating the relative importance of each criterion in the set. This weighting action takes into consideration that all criteria may not be of equal importance or bear equally on the decision.

The assignment of weights is best arrived at by rank ordering the relative importance of criteria in the set and then applying the weighting points, using judgment to arrive at the actual numbers. The group may use multivoting to facilitate rank ordering each criterion within the set. Figure 4-2 presents sample weighted decision criteria.

Several categories of decision criteria may be considered: key processes, organizational competencies, principal measures of performance, and issues of strategic importance to the collaborative. Each of these four areas is detailed in separate subsections.

Key Processes

In chapter 1, a key process was defined as those essential activities that must be performed optimally to meet customers' needs. Organizations can use key processes to focus their benchmarking efforts and help ensure development of superior performance in those areas that matter most to customers.

Key processes, which play a significant role in benchmarking and in quality initiatives, provide a context for managing these efforts and aiding in project selection. Not only do they offer a framework for resource allocation decisions, they represent the processes health care providers use to create their essential products and services.

An example of a key process for an acute care provider is case management. Within the case management macro process might lie subprocesses such

Figure 4-2. Sample Weighted Decision Criteria

Criteria	Weight
1. Have impact on costs across the system	25
2. Relate to key process of central office and affiliates	15
3. Relate to one of the strategies in the existing strategic plan	20
4. Have impact on all types of facilities	15
5. Relate to central office activity	5
6. Be seen as important issue by affiliates	12
7. Be "doable"	8

as certification and triage assessment, assessment and diagnosis, care and treatment planning, clinical intervention, and clinical outcomes evaluation. Another example is an organization's human resource management system, a macro process that might be further divided into recruiting and hiring, training and development, salary and benefits administration, performance management, payroll, and employee relations.

Because they are important contributors to quality initiatives and benchmarking, an organization must identify its key processes. Health care providers have applied several approaches to identifying key processes. Four of these approaches are a "top down–bottom up" method, borrowed from industry; adoption of key processes identified by the Joint Commission on Accreditation of Healthcare Organizations (JCAHO); a "walk-through" of customers' experiences; and the Organizing Work as a System method developed by the Quality Resource Center of the Hospital Corporation of America.

Using "Top Down–Bottom Up" Discussion

The "top down–bottom up" approach, used by companies such as Xerox, involves top management challenging middle management to identify key processes of the organization. Middle management in turn identifies a draft set of key processes, which top management reviews and modifies if necessary. Figure 4-3 lists key processes selected at Xerox using this discussion. Some health care organizations, among them Mercy Midlands, have also utilized this discussion approach to identify their key processes. (See figure 4-4.)

The chief advantage of the top down–bottom up method is the management team's commitment to the key processes developed as a result of its work. A second advantage is the fact that key processes are tailored to the unique needs of the organization.

A disadvantage of this approach is that no blueprint guides the discussions or development of key processes. Because of this lack of structure, the team may spend considerable time arriving at key processes. Another disadvantage is the difficulty organizations have in breaking out of the departmental mind-set. In those instances, the key processes identified follow departmental lines rather than reflecting cross-functional processes.

Adopting the Key Processes Identified by the JCAHO

Health care organizations may adopt the key processes identified by the JCAHO and shown in figure 4-5. The JCAHO terminology used to designate critical activities performed by health care organizations is *important functions*. One advantage of this approach lies primarily in identification of key processes actually performed and the thorough coverage this set provides. Another advantage by implication is the organization's preparation for future accreditation.

Figure 4-3. Business Processes Selected by Xerox

Market Management

- Market planning
- Product planning and development
- Pricing
- Market tracking
- Product life-cycle management
- Marketing communications

Customer Engagement

- Sales territory planning
- Prospecting management
- Enterprise management
- Agreement development
- Agreement management
- Customer support

Order Fulfillment

- Order processing
- Scheduling
- Customer preparation
- Staging and preinstallation
- Delivery/removal
- Installation/deinstallation
- Product production

Product Maintenance

- Service call management
- Service dispatching
- Product servicing
- Service call closure
- Product maintenance planning
- Equipment performance monitoring
- Technical information provision
- Service territory planning

Billing and Collection

- Invoicing
- Banking operations
- Cash application
- Collection
- Third-party leasing administration

Financial Management

- Financial planning
- Financial analysis and reporting
- Financial outlooking
- Tax planning and management
- Accounting operations
- Financial auditing
- Disbursements
- Financial asset/cash planning
- Financial asset control

Inventory Management and Logistics

- Physical asset acquisition
- Inventory management
- Physical asset planning
- Logistics planning
- Logistics operations
- Logistics engineering
- Vendor management

Business Management

- Business strategy development
- Business planning
- Business process and operations management
  - Process specification
  - Coordination and integration
  - Inspection
  - Benchmarking
  - Process improvement

Information Technology Management

- Information strategy planning
- Systems analysis and design
- Systems development
- Production systems support
- Research and development
- Business systems management coordination

Human Resource Management

- Manpower requirements planning
- Hiring and assignment
- Benefits and compensation management
- Personnel management
- Work force preparedness
- Employee communications

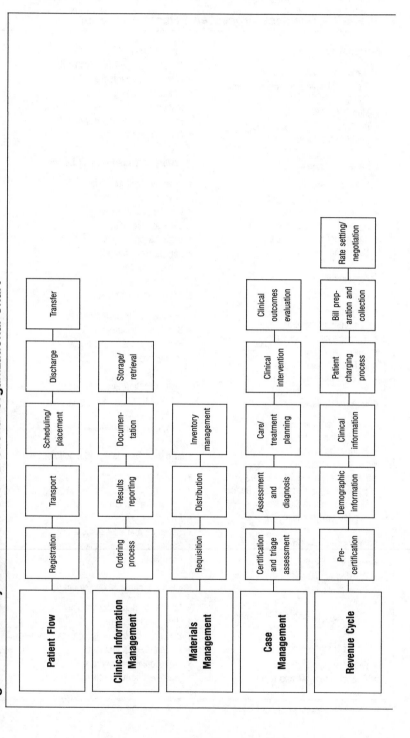

Figure 4-4. Mercy Midlands Cross-Functional Organizational Chart

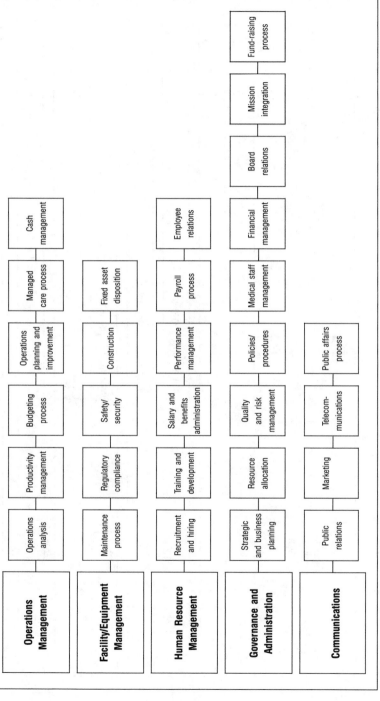

Figure 4-5. JCAHO Important Functions and Structures

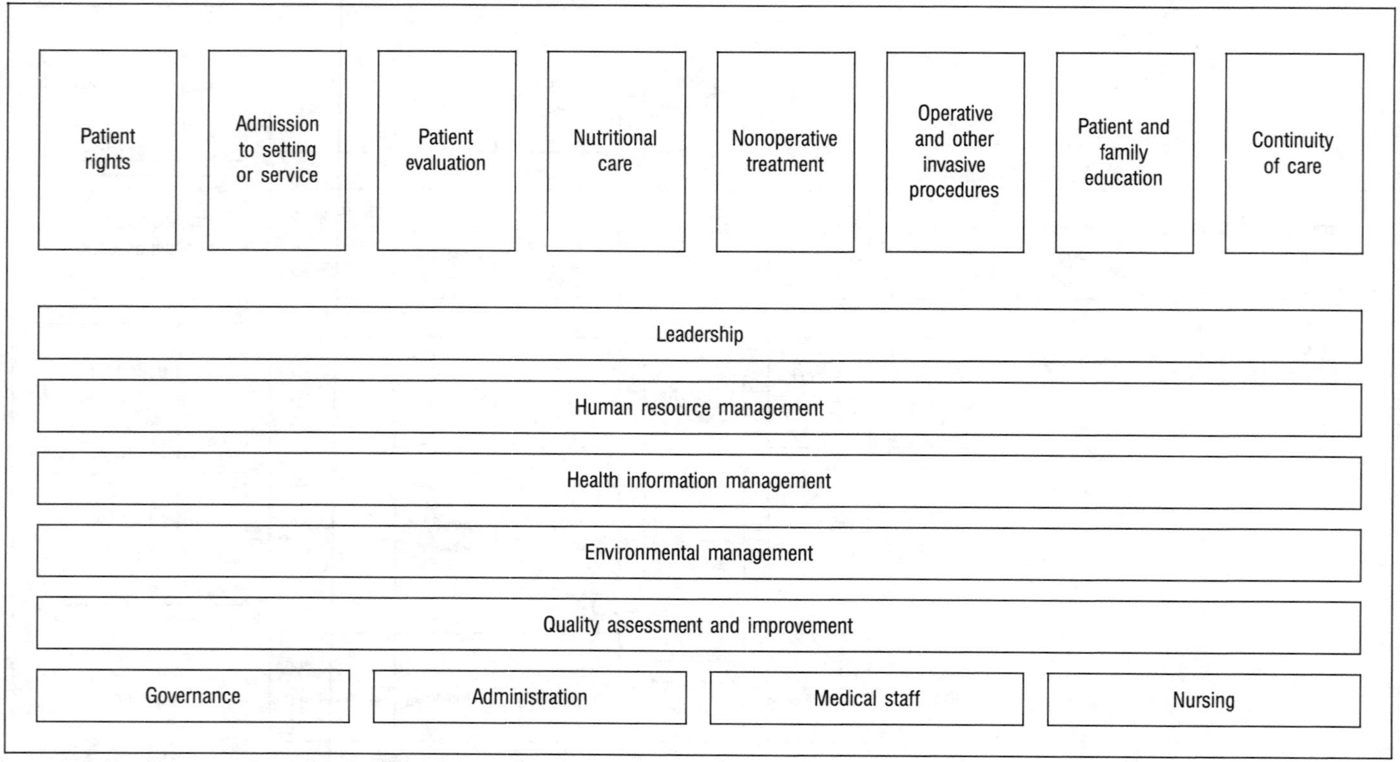

Reprinted, with permission, from the Joint Commission on Accreditation of Healthcare Organizations, copyright 1994.

A disadvantage of this approach is the generic nature of the set and its macro level. This means that if the group adopts key processes developed outside the organization, the implications of those processes may not be thoroughly understood internally. Furthermore, generic key processes may not reflect the functions important to a particular organization or its customers.

"Walking Through" the Customers' Experiences

In "walking through" the experiences of customers (inpatients, outpatients, and emergency patients for example), senior managers discuss major systems customers interact with when dealing with the organization. This discussion may be unstructured and may take place away from the actual activities where services are provided. Or, senior leaders may physically walk through the steps experienced by customers while being served. In either case the team constructs a set of key processes encountered by customers and identifies the supporting subprocesses. An example of key processes resulting from this walk-through approach as used at St. John's Regional Medical Center is presented in figure 4-6.

Several advantages recommend this approach. First, the development team will use the set for decision making about benchmarking and improvement projects. Again, like key processes that emerge from top down–bottom up discussion, a walk-through set reflects the specific needs of the organization. There is also the group insight and acceptance through ownership gained from developing the set.

The chief disadvantage of this approach is limited knowledge of customer experience on the part of participants who use the set. Again, a departmental rather than a cross-functional orientation can result due to the historical mind-set of participants.

Organizing Work as a System

The Quality Resource Center of the Hospital Corporation of America developed an approach that lends itself to identifying key processes.[3] This method was originally designed as a learning exercise to help participants develop an overview of organizational activities and an appreciation for the systemic nature of those activities. The team in this instance is comprised of senior leaders. This exercise may be conducted for the health care organization as a whole or for specific departments. For the purposes of identifying key processes, the exercise is applied to the total organization.

This approach uses the series of structured discussion questions, listed in figure 4-7, that lead to an understanding of how the organization works as a system. The answers disclose the core work system of the health care organization. Within that system, participants identify key processes used to produce the products and services created by the organization.

Figure 4-6.   SJRMC Core Systems

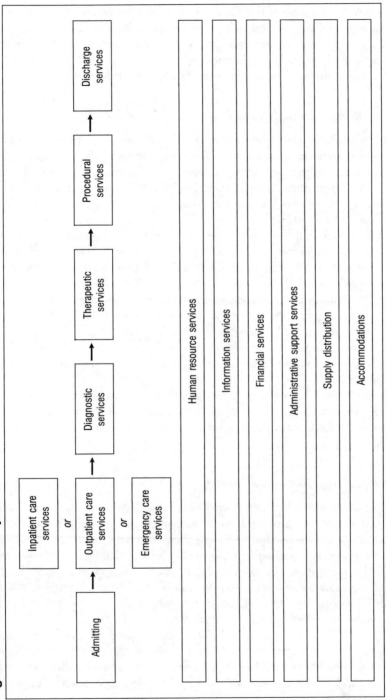

Figure 4-7. Organizing Work as a System

1. What do we produce?

2. Who uses or receives what we make?

3. What is the underlying need that those customers have for what we produce?

4. What characteristics do customers use when they assess and judge the goodness or quality of what we make? What about customers might prompt or drive their interest in assessing and judging quality that way?

5. What methods do we use to accomplish what we produce?

6. What comes into our process and is changed by or used within the actions of the process to create the products or services?

7. Who or what specific people, departments, or organizations provide the inputs?

8. Based on what we know about the need for what we do, and our knowledge of the customers, what is the aim for the future in our organization?

9. Based on our aim for the future, on our knowledge of the customer, on information from employees involved, and on knowledge about our work, what is strategically important to improve?

10. What specific processes offer us the greatest leverage in securing the strategic improvements we seek?

For example, responses to question 1, What do we produce? might be procedures, information, reports, decisions, therapeutic services, or a conducive environment. Procedures might include laboratory tests, radiology exams, and surgical interventions. A conducive environment includes the physical space as well as the organizational culture.

The question most relevant for the purposes of this discussion is question 5, What methods do we use to accomplish what we produce? In enumerating the processes or activities that yield the products answered in question 1, this list can become quite long. Once arranged in a logical sequence, however, these processes can reflect a typical scenario of what happens as a patient is moved through the system. Several of these processes come together to form key processes within the organization. For example, key processes of a health care provider might include (but not be limited to) acquiring new patients, admitting patients, assessing patient needs, delivering services, and evaluating services. Other processes (subprocesses) support these key processes. Support processes for registering patients might include scheduling, verifying financial and demographic information, verifying insurance information, and seeking credit approval. (Remember, key processes for health care providers are those that further the customer care.)

This systematic approach progresses logically from question to question, a primary advantage of this method. It can be used to identify both key and subordinate processes while participants gain understanding of the organization as a system. Figure 4-8 shows a sample exercise that promotes understanding the systemic relationships within an organization.

Figure 4-8. Organizing Work as a System (Exercise)

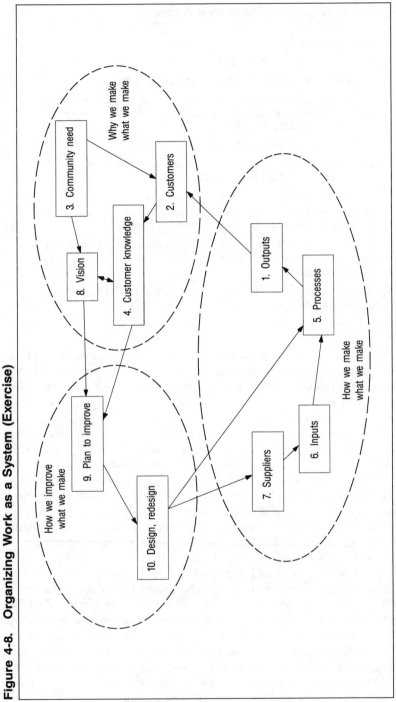

The Organizing Work as a System method requires a disciplined team willing to commit time to complete the complex exercise. In addition, some questions may need verification of the initial responses with customer data, another time investment.

Because health care organizations will ultimately form the collaborative, those organizations likely have similar key processes. These key processes, and the sample methods for arriving at them as described above, can be used to identify candidates for benchmarking projects, as well as criteria for selection.

Organizational Competencies

Organizational competencies represent another category of criteria used to select benchmarking projects. Competencies may be defined as what a company is especially good at or, more important, how well a company applies know-how in offering products and services. Instead of the typically static question What business are we really in? Tomasko advises organizations to probe more deeply by asking What special skills and know-how do we bring to the businesses we are now in that can serve as a foundation upon which future businesses can be built?[4]

Watson encourages selecting the competencies that matter, recognizing that all competencies are not equal.[5] Organizations must identify their competencies, segregate them, and improve the ones that really count. Figure 4-9 delineates four types of competencies and their relative importance, a categorization scheme devised by Tomasko. Each type is discussed below.

Cutting-Edge Competencies

Cutting-edge competencies represent the source of tomorrow's success. These competencies, which prove most crucial to meeting the future needs of customers, must be embedded in future products and services an organization provides. According to an article in the *Harvard Business Review*, "An organization's capacity to improve existing skills and learn new ones is the most defensible

Figure 4-9. Organizational Competencies

Type	Role
Cutting edge	Source of tomorrow's competitiveness
Critical	Source of today's competitive advantage
Core	Common to most businesses in the same industry
Complementary	Support services, internal competencies

Reprinted, with permission, from *Rethinking the Corporation,* published by AMACOM, New York, NY, copyright 1993.

competitive advantage of all."[6] The ability of Magic Valley Medical Center (Twin Falls, Idaho) to transform its orientation from an inpatient, internal acute care focus to a wellness, healthier community focus demonstrates a cutting-edge competency in that it foretells the facility's capacity to continue anticipating customer demands. By targeting critical competencies for benchmarking, organizations can better position themselves for future success.

Critical Competencies

Critical competencies separate one organization from another and define why customers prefer the novelty and uniqueness of one organization or product over another. Critical competencies represent the source of today's success and provide opportunities for growth. Examples of critical competencies include cancer care at M. D. Anderson Medical Center (Houston, Texas) or the holistic care provided by Mid Columbia Hospital (The Dalles, Oregon). Benchmarking critical competencies allows organizations to improve their standing in current markets.

Core Competencies

Core competencies include those common to most organizations within a particular industry. Generally, customers cannot differentiate core competencies from one organization to another, but they may notice their absence. Regarding them as basic to organizational performance, customers accept them as a matter of course. Delivering inpatient nursing care for acute care hospitals or completing a telephone call for a communications company exemplify core competencies. Core competencies make good candidates for benchmarking within an organization's own industry but can, by this same narrowness, limit opportunities for true breakthrough improvements.

Complementary Competencies

Complementary competencies are those mostly associated with support services, the work behind the scenes. Their low visibility may also make them least important to customers. Within health care organizations, cost for complementary competencies such as administrative support personnel, materials management, or accounting represents the most important critical success factor. Fledgling benchmarking health care organizations may target these types of competencies, since they are most common among potential benchmarking partners in other industries. The downside is that complementary competencies may not lift overall organizational performance to needed levels and that improvements may not be readily apparent to customers.

A common thread in these four types of organizational competencies is competitive strength in relation to customer needs. Because customer needs do not remain static, nor can competencies. In the context of benchmarking, competencies can be learned and improved over time.

Finally, competencies require a blend of processes to produce the desired effect—customer satisfaction. For example, a health care provider perceived to be patient friendly to patients and to provide excellent patient service has a competency that results from several human resources processes. These processes include hiring and training of employees, employee relations, and internal communications.[7] Competencies provide an effective criterion base for selecting benchmarking projects and help ensure that an organization's benchmarking efforts focus on issues important to achieving customer satisfaction.

Principal Measures of Performance

Principal measures of performance, also called key indicators, critical success factors, leading operational indicators, or key results areas, can help determine significance of outcomes. Spendolini defines principal measures as "subjects significant enough to warrant the use of benchmarking."[8] Rockart regards them as the "limited number of areas in which results, if they are satisfactory, will ensure successful competitive performance for the organization."[9] Principal measures of performance may be classified broadly into three groups—quality, time, and cost.

In terms of quality, principal measures of performance for health care organizations include, for example, patient satisfaction ratings and positive patient outcomes. Those measures relating to time include average length of stay for selected patient populations (a specific diagnosis-related group or a particular managed care contract) and the cycle time for an important issue, such as days in accounts receivable. Cost-based principal measures of performance, which may be the most prevalent indicator in many health care organizations today, include cost per adjusted patient day, operating margin, and labor cost as a percentage of total operating expenses (among others).

The challenge for most organizations is to identify principal measures of performance that relate to *meaningful and desired* organizational results, not simply those that are convenient or required. Ideally these measures should be linked to the key processes that produce desired results. In this way, organizations gain meaningful measures of both results and process.

Significant work is being conducted in outcomes measurement. An example of such research, and the resulting indicators that might represent principal measures of performance, is demonstrated by the Consortium Research on Indicators of System Performance (CRISP). CRISP is working to identify measures of overall performance of a health care system. Figure 4-10 shows the 12 initial indicators created by the Consortium.[10]

Strategically Important Issues

As indicated by the opening quotation to this chapter, what is benchmarked should be strategically important in terms of what it takes to accomplish the

Figure 4-10.   CRISP Indicators

• Service quality/access 　—Patient satisfaction	• Prevention/screening 　—Prevention index
• Appropriateness 　—Admissions per member per year 　—Days per 1,000 member per year 　—Utilization rates	• Enrollee health 　—Functional status measure—SF36 • Financial performance 　—Debt service coverage
• Sophisticated clinical 　—Readmission rate 　—Low birthweight incidence rate	—Percent system expenses for administration 　—Profitability 　—Portion of system expenses devoted to charity

Reprinted, with permission, from the Center for Health Systems Studies, Henry Ford Health System, copyright 1993.

desired outcomes. Benchmarking provides a means of accelerating the achievement of organizational strategy. To maximize this effort, the organization may consider its mission, values, vision, and strategic direction in selecting benchmarking projects. Doing so ensures that the selection process reinforces alignment of the organization's actions with its beliefs. Such consistency between resource utilization and strategic intent also allows issues to be supported strategically with meaningful action.

The Aluminum Company of America (ALCOA) stresses the importance of strategy, mission, and values in its six-step approach to benchmarking. To ensure the relevancy and validity of project selection, sponsors must answer the question "Is the topic consistent with ALCOA's mission, values, and milestones?"[11] Health care leaders faced with selecting benchmarking projects would be well advised to answer the same question.

Issues of strategic importance provide excellent candidates for benchmarking projects. Ideally, strategic priorities should incorporate organizational competencies, key processes, and be monitored by principal measures of performance so as to justify being the focus of breakthrough improvement initiatives. For example, a health care organization's strategic initiative to focus on emergency care in its marketplace is driven by the forces of the market. To excel at providing emergency services, the organization may elect to benchmark aspects of its emergency care delivery (such as patient wait time) with those of other health care providers outside its market. Or it can compare its performance with other industries that deal with on-demand, high-turnaround activities. On-demand, high-turnaround activities include any type of queueing—waiting line—functions, such as fast food restaurants, grocery stores, and hotel registrations.

Other Considerations

Although these four categories of criteria—key processes, competencies, principal measures, and key strategic issues—provide good bases for selecting benchmarking projects, others are equally useful so long as they reflect the conditions individual organizations want their benchmarking efforts to meet. For example, criteria such as amount of time estimated to undertake the project, potential scope of the topic, geographic locations, or project applicability and/or impact on type of facility or on the kind of care provided (acute or long-term) all are valid considerations.

As this chapter makes clear, a vast pool of decision criteria can be drawn on for topic selection. One multifacility health care system that launched a benchmarking project for which (after months of formal and informal discussions among staff) the following seven criteria were developed:

1. Have impact on costs across the system
2. Relate to key process of central office and affiliates
3. Relate to one of the strategies in the existing strategic plan
4. Have impact on all types of facilities
5. Relate to central office activity
6. Be seen as important issue by affiliates
7. Be "doable"

Step 2: Generate List of Potential Study Topics

Health care organizations abound with opportunities for breakthrough improvement that lend themselves to benchmarking projects. These opportunities (topics) may come from several sources including customer feedback, strategically important issues, and staff suggestions.

Customer Feedback

Given that a primary purpose of benchmarking is to achieve breakthrough improvement in meeting customer expectations, it follows that customer feedback is an excellent source for potential projects. For example, routine comments about service delays in a particular department might trigger project identification, as might patterns of failure to meet customer expectations. Poor survey scores and patient reports also help identify areas of opportunity. Gathering this kind of data implies that organizations must have information systems in place to facilitate data collection and analysis about customers, their requirements, and event reports of instances where those requirements have not been met. Satisfaction surveys and questionnaires, phone follow-up, patient population profiles, and patient education programs are only some of the feedback tools available for this purpose.

Strategic Issues

As discussed earlier in the chapter, a strategic focus entails increased likelihood for significant organizational improvements. The emergency services example given earlier in the chapter represents an opportunity that can be added to the list of prospects. A strategic thrust to become the most cost-effective tertiary care provider in its region is another. Particular projects within this latter strategy might include benchmarking to compare cost and length of stay with other providers (locally or nationwide) or studying support service provision with that of other health care facilities or non-health care industries to identify better methods (for example patient relations and customer service).

Staff Suggestions

Staff members have first-hand knowledge of customers and their needs and can provide a rich source for benchmarking project ideas. Topics such as radiology turnaround time, total joint replacement, and foodservice delivery are some examples. Staff not involved in direct patient care might suggest projects on time required to fill vacancies, days in accounts receivable, and high-cost/low-profitability DRGs. These topics tend to be operations focused and therefore can provide opportunity to improve service and performance.

There should be no fear of having too few projects from which to choose. On the contrary, the "problem" may lie in having too many. The health system that identified the decision criteria in the previous section also created the following list of potential benchmarking projects:

- High-cost DRGs
- Low-profitability DRGs
- DRGs with long lengths of stay
- Product standardization
- Number of X rays taken
- Workers' compensation
- Acuity systems and staffing
- Utilization review
- Medical staff credentialing
- Days in accounts receivable
- Foodservice operations in residential housing

The projects on the list are a result of a series of discussions among the system management team, ideas from team conversations with facility management, and suggestions from staff.

Step 3: Apply Decision Criteria

Having identified selection criteria as described earlier in the chapter—key processes, organizational competencies, performance measures, and strategic intent—the team now must find a way to reach consensus on a benchmarking project. To maximize active participation of other organizations that may be involved in the effort, the sponsoring organization must choose a project that is sufficiently important to warrant that involvement.

First the list of potential candidates must be shortened as necessary to those few deserving further consideration. Decision theory provides a tool used frequently in quality management—the decision matrix.[12] A decision matrix permits multiple criteria to be considered in making a complex decision. The sample decision matrix shown in figure 4-11 is constructed on the list of potential projects listed above. The tool lists all criteria involved in the decision (top), their numeric relative importance (or weights), and all projects under consideration (left-hand column).

The decision makers next rate each candidate project, typically on a scale from 1 to 3 with 1 being low; 2, medium; and 3, high. Other scales can range from 1 to 7. The difficulty with a broader scale is inability to differentiate clearly between the rating levels, which can skew matrix results.

Two other options may be used to score the decision matrix and eliminate potential projects. In the first, decision makers rate alternatives independently and then convene to compile their aggregate scores and resolve major differences among individual scores.

In the second option, the group discusses and scores the decision matrix as a group. The benefit here is that discussion and resolution of differences among individual scores takes place in only one session.

Both methods are effective, and the selection of one over the other rests primarily with the comfort group's level. The matrix is a tool, not a replacement for decision making. Also, decision makers must rate each proposed project solely according to the criteria identified earlier and included on the tool. The rating given each potential project for each decision criterion is then multiplied by the respective weight of that criterion. These weighted ratings are then summed to compute the total score for the alternative.

A completed decision matrix is shown in figure 4-12. The number of candidates was reduced from 11 to 2—workers' compensation (280 points) and days in accounts receivable (260 points)—reflecting the two highest scores from the decision matrix. The gap between these two and the third candidate (acuity systems and staffing, 225 points) was felt to be wide enough to limit further discussion.

Before applying the decision matrix, the management team in this example spent considerable time discussing the relative merits of each candidate project in an unstructured way. Once the matrix was used, the list was pared down and more focused discussion ensued. Again, the purpose of applying the decision matrix is to reduce the number of options, not to select the project.

Step 4: Agree on Project Selection

Once the group reduces the number of potential benchmarking projects to a manageable number (typically four or fewer, assuming one project will be

Figure 4-11. Sample Decision Matrix

Decision Criteria →	Cost	Key Process	Strategy	All Facility Types	Central Office Activity	Important	Doable	Total Score
Candidate Project Weights →	25	15	20	15	5	12	8	
High-cost DRGs								
Low-profit DRGs								
DRGs with long lengths of stay								
Product standardization								
Number of X rays taken								
Workers' compensation								
Acuity systems and staffing								
Utilization review								
Medical staff credentialing								
Days in accounts receivable								
Food service in residential housing								

Figure 4-12. Sample Completed Decision Matrix

Decision Criteria → Candidate Project	Cost	Key Process	Strategy	All Facility Types	Central Office Activity	Important	Doable	Total Score
Weights →	25	15	20	15	5	12	8	
High-cost DRGs	3	2	2	1	1	2	2	205
Low-profit DRGs	3	2	2	1	1	2	2	205
DRGs with long lengths of stay	3	2	2	1	1	2	2	205
Product standardization	2	1	1	2	1	1	2	148
Number of X rays taken	1	1	1	1	1	1	2	113
Workers' compensation	3	3	2	3	3	3	3	280
Acuity systems and staffing	3	2	1	2	2	3	2	225
Utilization review	2	1	1	1	1	1	1	125
Medical staff credentialing	1	1	1	1	1	1	2	108
Days in accounts receivable	3	3	2	3	3	3	3	260
Food service in residential housing	1	2	1	1	1	2	3	143

launched), the remaining candidates can be evaluated more closely to arrive at final project selection. The same decision criteria identified previously can be used to guide the discussion. The candidates need not be scored again, although it is important to underscore the need for consensus in the final project selection, as unanimity will drive leaders' support for execution of the project.

This less-structured final project discussion acknowledges the advantages and disadvantages of each potential project. In addition, each decision maker's insight on the issues is shared to ensure that the objective analysis of the decision matrix is blended with the benefits of more personal group discussion. The team revisited the decision criteria used to screen the proposed project list as well as considered recent performance improvements in the candidate processes. The trend in days in accounts receivable was favorable, and had been in recent years. Comparative data indicated that, while improvement was still possible, performance was better than in other systems. The trend in workers' compensation costs had shown improvement, but recent signs showed a return to old performance levels. The group also discussed the visibility of the project to affiliated facilities. Given these comparisons, final agreement was to benchmark workers' compensation.

Summary

Selecting the right project to benchmark is a key ingredient for project success. Factors such as time and money expenditure, among others, help determine which benchmarking projects to undertake. Organizations can combine objective analysis with unstructured group discussion to increase the likelihood of selecting the right project. By first identifying criteria for project selection (using key processes, competencies, strategic issues, and principal performance indicators, among others), leaders can generate a list of possible topics. After streamlining the list and arriving at a final consensus agreement, a project can be launched.

Putting These Ideas to Work

Objective

Identify possible candidates from which to select an initial benchmarking project at your organization.

Approach

1. Brainstorm a list of possible criteria for project selection.
2. Combine entries that might be duplicates.
3. Prioritize entries using multivoting or rank ordering.
4. Select the most important entries on the list, anywhere from five to eight.

5. Assign weights to the entries by dividing the number of entries by 100, giving more points to those entries you deem more important.
6. Audit the list to be sure it is consistent with how you feel about the entries and their respective weights.
7. The resulting list represents the decision criteria you would use to select a benchmarking project from those proposed.
8. Brainstorm a list of possible candidates for benchmarking projects in your organization.
9. Define each candidate project sufficiently to allow for discussion.
10. Eliminate candidates that obviously are in opposition to the criteria developed.
11. Apply the criteria to the remaining candidates on the list.
12. Use the individual ratings and weights to calculate scores for the candidates.
13. Discuss candidates that score highest and then select from them.

References and Notes

1. C. Jackson Grayson, quoted in Healthcare organizations adapt benchmarking techniques from industry to make gains. *The Quality Letter*, Sept. 1992, p. 6.

2. Juran, J. M. Universals in management planning and control. *The Management Review* 43(11):748–61, Nov. 1954.

3. Quality Resource Group, Hospital Corporation of America. *Organizing Work as a System*. Unpublished work. Nashville, TN: Hospital Corporation of America, July 15, 1992.

4. Tomasko, R. M. *Rethinking the Corporation*. New York City: AMACOM, 1993, pp. 37–38.

5. Watson, G. H. *The Benchmarking Workbook: Adapting Best Practices for Performance Improvement*. Cambridge, MA: Productivity Press, 1992, p. 21.

6. Prahalad, C. K., and Hamel, G. Strategic intent. *Harvard Business Review* 67(3):68, May–June, 1989.

7. Example, adapted from Tomasko, R. M. *Rethinking the Corporation*. New York City: AMACOM, 1993, p. 43.

8. Spendolini, M. J. *The Benchmarking Book*. New York City: AMACOM, 1992, p. 68.

9. Rockart, J. F. Chief executive officers define their own data needs. *Harvard Business Review* 57(2):81–93, Mar.–Apr. 1979.

10. Health Care Advisory Board. *Outcomes Sourcebook: Profiles of Leading Tracking Systems*. Washington, DC: Advisory Board Company, 1993, pp. 40–41.

11. Benowski, K. The benchmarking bandwagon. *Quality Progress* 24(1):22, Jan. 1991.

12. For a more detailed review of the application of a decision matrix, refer to Wendy Leebov and Clara Jean Ersoz, eds. *The Health Care Manager's Guide to Continuous Quality Improvement*. Chicago: American Hospital Publishing, 1991, pp. 169–73.

Phase 2: Form the Collaborative

Introduction

To carry out the collaborative approach recommended in this book, organizations work cooperatively to facilitate development of relationships that focus attention not only on the project but on the group that structures those working relationships. This group is referred to as the *benchmarking collaborative*, comprised of those representatives from participant organizations that come together to conduct the benchmarking project. The collaborative plays a critical role in the project's success and must be assembled with careful attention.

The collaborative determines ground rules for participation and conduct and serves as a decision-making body. It may set up a *guidance team* to provide functional supervision of the project and to interact with the discrete *benchmarking teams* at participating organizations. The decision whether to appoint a guidance team depends in part on the number of organizations participating in the project.

The size of a benchmarking collaborative dictates how it is structured. A small group (15 or fewer participants) may operate without a guidance team. A group of more than 15, however, may form a guidance team that is a subset of members of the benchmarking collaborative. The guidance team operates much like a *quality council* in that it creates ground rules to govern how it will operate; that is, it identifies criteria for decision making and relies on consensus approval of group actions from its members. The element of consensus building—gaining understanding and acceptance of actions before continuing—is key to project success and future collaboration.

The following two examples illustrate how a collaborative might be structured. Six facilities within a multifacility health system came together to study and improve organizational performance in early return to work programs. That effort was coordinated by five staff from the central office. These staff members plus one representative from each participating facility formed the 11-member benchmarking collaborative for this project.

Twelve facilities in another multifacility health system studied medication errors. This effort was supported by five staff from the corporate office. One representative from each facility and the five corporate staff comprise the benchmarking collaborative. These 17 individuals believed the group too large to function effectively and created a guidance team to coordinate the project.

Structure of the collaborative also depends on how familiar participants are with each other and on how much previous experience they have with working collaboratively. As trust increases, members may feel more comfortable turning over project control to a guidance team. Figure 5-1 is a schematic representation of these relationships, which are addressed in more detail later in the chapter.

This chapter describes nine steps for establishing a benchmarking collaborative:

1. Determine interest in forming a collaborative.
2. Identify potential participant organizations.
3. Identify key decision makers.
4. Explore and generate interest in project and collaborative.
5. Confirm participants' level of interest.
6. Identify and educate stakeholders.
7. Create a collaborative project charter.
8. Adopt a benchmarking ethics code.
9. Initiate the project and select a guidance team.

Figure 5-2 presents a flowchart of the general approach to setting up a benchmarking collaborative. This approach proceeds from the spark of interest generated by the sponsoring group through launching the project.

Step 1: Determine Interest in Forming a Collaborative

Typically the idea to conduct a benchmarking project stems from an individual (project champion) or an organization (sponsoring organization). As mentioned in chapter 3, before setting out to establish the collaborative, the sponsoring organization already will have determined the topic of the benchmarking effort. Although topic details may not be fully known, the champion or sponsoring organization must have a subject in which sufficient interest in launching a project can be gauged.

The project champion must be articulate enough to explain the rationale for the project, to communicate effectively in groups and individually, and to make the case for both the project and the collaborative. This individual must describe benefits that potential participating organizations will receive from participating collaboratively in the benchmarking project. To accomplish these purposes, the champion must be seen as credible and competent in order to give the project legitimacy in the organization.

Figure 5-1. Sample Structure of a Benchmarking Collaborative

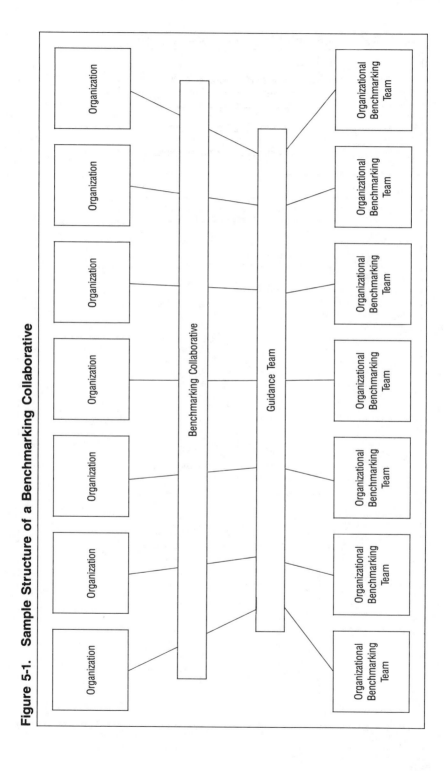

Figure 5-2.   Establish the Benchmarking Collaborative

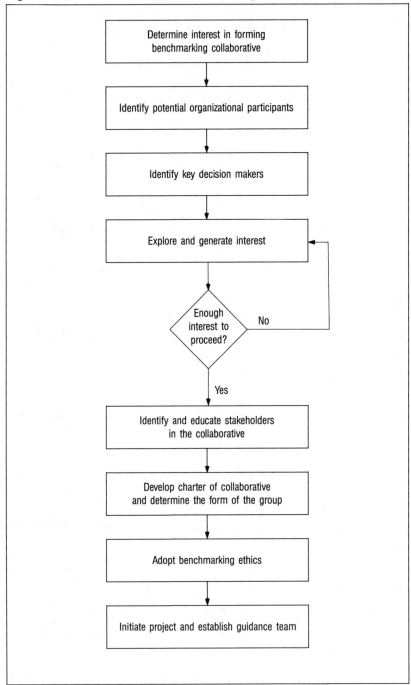

Supporting characteristics of this function include project management skills and consultative skills. Coordinating development of the benchmarking collaborative requires managerial ability to synchronize the agendas of multiple organizations toward one end—initiation of the benchmarking project. Consultative skills are essential because the collaborative functions as a loose-knit group, with little or no direct control.

The project champion role may be shared by anyone advocating project selection and launch. In fact, the broader the base of advocacy the greater the likelihood of success. In practice, championing the benchmarking project is almost always a group effort in that once conceived and endorsed, the project thrives on group effort to demonstrate benefits of the project to other potential participant organizations. Such effort requires the time and talents of multiple people, all of whom become project champions.

To determine the level of interest, the project champion or sponsor must first convey to senior leaders within the organization the benefits expected from conducting the project. The champion must also underscore advantages of conducting the project in a collaborative manner. Two key advantages are increased potential for learning and cost effectiveness of this approach to benchmarking studies.

A critical factor in generating interest lies in comparing benefits to be derived from the project with costs incurred in conducting it. The collaborative model provides a cost-effective vehicle for learning that improves organizational performance. The alternatives are either to forgo a benchmarking study or for a single organization to conduct the study, incurring all risks and costs singlehandedly.

Step 2: Identify Potential Participant Organizations

Once the organization is satisfied that there is sufficient interest in conducting a collaborative benchmarking project, the next step is to identify potential participant organizations. This task is easier if the organization is part of a health system, alliance, or network than if it is a freestanding entity. Stand-alone organizations face the most difficulty in this area and may need to work with local, regional, or state associations. (More will be said on affiliated versus nonaffiliated facilities later in this section.)

The size of the prospective collaborative is another factor in identifying participants. A collaborative may range anywhere from 2 to as many as 35 organizations, as in The Healthcare Forum's benchmarking study into inpatient elective admitting practices in 1992. The size of a collaborative is directly proportional to complexity of the effort, and although no rigid rules apply here, between 6 and 10 participants appears most workable.

Typically, one representative from each participating organization sits as a member of the collaborative. In addition, the collaborative may choose to supplement its resources with specialty staff from participating organizations. Often, the sponsoring organization provides these specialty staff, who might include experts in benchmarking mechanics, survey designers, or trainers, making for a pretty sizable collaborative.

There may be a trade-off between group size and diversity. Whereas a smaller group might operate more effectively, it may not provide as many opportunities for participants to learn from each other as a large one might. This limitation may not be solely a function of number of participants. For example, a well-structured collaborative will be made up of participants that differ in size, location, and service mix—depending on the topic being studied. If the collaborative is studying coronary artery bypass grafts, obviously it cannot include facilities that do not perform that procedure, unless it is studying support or administrative processes connected with that surgical intervention. The broader the base of participants, the more opportunities there are for learning. Conversely, if membership is monolithic, performing the same processes in exactly the same ways, little chance exists for learning.

In identifying possible participants for the workers' compensation study, planners sought a mix of experts in workers' compensation. Representatives from finance, risk management, employee health, human resources, safety, patient care services, and management were approached, as was an occupational health physician. This representation provided appropriate oversight to the activities of benchmarking teams in participating facilities. Members from the risk management and quality improvement departments in the central office served as support staff to the collaborative.

Affiliated Organizations

As stated above, size of the benchmarking collaborative may be affected by whether the organization is already affiliated. A collaborative composed of members of an existing system, alliance, consortium, or network has certain advantages. First, relationships, regardless of degree of formality, already exist, thus minimizing the time required for developing connections. A sense of history is in place, as are a shared vision and common group purpose. This in turn leads to easier project planning. A second advantage relates to size. Benchmarking collaboratives formed from existing groups may be larger than those created from stand-alone organizations. This may translate into more experience within the group and lower overall costs for each participant.

However, affiliated institutions face unique challenges. The very familiarity that joins the group can create barriers to moving forward, one of which is traditional cultural issues of the organization. For example, if the culture historically has focused on top–down control, the group may have trouble changing that focus to a more participatory approach that focuses on process as well as results. The collaborative must understand the diverse cultural issues among participant organizations and address those that impinge on the group's ability to function.

Stand-Alone Organizations

An organization that does not belong to an existing system, alliance, network, or consortium also brings certain advantages and challenges to the effort. The most significant advantage is enhanced flexibility in selecting participants. Given that participants are selected based on the project topic, the organization is unencumbered by broader considerations of standing or previous relationships. This permits selecting members that most desire active participation. Another advantage deals with the possible lack of long-standing relationships among participants. Just as an established relationship can propel the effort forward, absence of familiarity allows members to begin with a clean slate and without historical biases.

Absence of history also poses a challenge in terms of knowing how to identify the appropriate contacts so as to determine interest, willingness, and ability to participate. The time demands on a stand-alone entity seeking to form a collaborative may be formidable *because of* the period required to build trust among newly acquainted parties. Therefore, a benchmarking collaborative of strangers must devote more time and attention to teamship building.

Forming benchmarking collaboratives among known contacts is recommended as an accelerator in designing, conducting, and completing the project. These contacts include local, regional, or state health care associations, professional societies, and special-interest groups. In addition, purchasing cooperatives and vendors may provide a source of possible participants. An example referred to throughout the chapter is an insurance broker for a health system that provides a list of possible health care facility participants for inclusion in a benchmarking study of workers' compensation.

Step 3: Identify Key Decision Makers

The most significant success factor for the benchmarking collaborative is leadership support from participating organizations. Therefore, the chief executive officer and senior leadership team represent key decision makers. Their vision, communication, and actions determine the level of attention and acceptance the benchmarking project receives, within each participating organization and within the collaborative. Both attention and acceptance have strong bearing on the resources committed to study of the topic.

In addition, the middle manager who most "owns" the project or topic under study should be considered a key decision maker. The support and enthusiasm shown by this individual will contribute significantly to the organization's participation.

Identifying key decision makers depends on the status of potential participants in the collaborative. If the study is being conducted within the context of an existing structure (health system, alliance, consortium, or network), the task may be simplified by using directories to single out the organization's CEO, senior leadership teams, and middle management.

For organizations creating a benchmarking collaborative outside the context of existing structures, identifying key decision makers need not be difficult. The sources that helped the sponsoring organization identify potential participants provide opportunities for identifying key decision makers as well. Directories such as the *American Hospital Association Guide to the Health Care Field* provide specific information about health care facilities, including the names of CEOs. In addition, professional societies publish membership directories that generally include key personnel appropriate to the benchmarking project being proposed.

An informal source for key decision makers is the organization's staff and routine networking among health care professionals. Generally speaking, health care managers are fairly up-to-date on who their counterparts are in other organizations, which makes them a viable source for targeting key decision makers.

In the workers' compensation benchmarking example, key decision makers were identified from several sources. Because the project was conducted within a health system, the most readily available source was the directory of facility senior leadership teams. Developed and maintained by the central office, this directory provided the names and telephone numbers of its chief executive officers. Those responsible for risk management were identified through personal contacts with central office personnel.

Step 4: Explore and Generate Interest in Project and Collaborative

Securing commitment from leaders in participating organizations is crucial, and it requires building a sense of legitimacy of purpose for the project. Because so many challenges compete for the attention of health care leaders, benchmarking as a discipline and the benchmarking collaborative must prove their potential to resolve more issues than they create. Before they can sanction participation in the benchmarking collaborative, leaders must be convinced of efficacy of the approach and benefits of participation. Champions of the benchmarking cause must provide the information that promotes this understanding.

Building momentum for the project relies on learning where the sources of support and resistance lie. The benchmarking project champion and supporters can identify behaviors that range from excited anticipation to staunch opposition by conducting a force-field analysis. With this technique, participants identify two sets of forces: those motivating the organization to move from its current state to its desired future state and those restraining the organization from achieving its desired state. Listing these forces helps project supporters identify what issues they can leverage to gain support for the project in potential participating organizations. These "leverage points" allow supporters to build legitimacy for the project in the eyes of key decision makers. In addition, listing the restraining forces helps project supporters identify what barriers they must overcome to gain acceptance from key decision makers.

A force-field analysis may be constructed in any one of three ways. One, project supporters in the sponsoring organization may create a generic analysis, speculating on the issues that confront potential participants. This approach allows for a generalized set of forces to be identified rather quickly. It lacks, however, the specific issues each potential participating organization faces. The risk exists that the project champion may face a barrier posed by a potential participating organization that was not anticipated. Two, supporters can engage potential participants in its development. This might be done by approaching one organization at a time, possibly during project discussion. This second approach ensures that organization-specific issues will be disclosed. The risk, however, is that the project sponsor may not be able to respond to any restraining forces raised. Three, an amalgam of the two preceding options involves the project sponsor's creation of a generic force-field analysis to prepare for discussions with potential participants, who may or may not be told an analysis is under way. During those discussions, the project sponsor could engage key decision makers in amending the analysis to fit their specific situations. In this way, both contingencies (acceptance or rejection) are considered. An example of a force-field analysis conducted for the workers' compensation benchmarking study is shown in figure 5-3.

Figure 5-3. Workers' Compensation Force-Field Analysis

Driving Forces	Restraining Forces
Reduce facility costs	No buy-in on WC as an issue
Improve continuity of care	Resistance to corporate idea
Reduce harm to employees	Time
Improve organizational productivity	Cost
Improve staff morale	Resources
Improve WC system efficiency	Resistance to change
Meet regulatory requirements	Lack of discipline
Increase awareness	Lack of incentive
Create best practices model	Geographic dispersion
Increase knowledge of scope of problem	Differing state statutes
Reduce facility risk	Skills
Improve service to facilities	Complacency
	Lack of measurement
	Data inconsistency

Step 5: Confirm Participants' Level of Interest

Once the level of interest among potential participants is ascertained, project champions and supporters must determine if that interest is sufficient to proceed. Have enough organizations committed so that the benchmarking effort will be cost effective *and* successful? No algorithm can quantify "enough organizations." Rather, that determination must be made based simply on the number of organizations that indicate interest. Discussions to arrive at consensus to proceed with a collaborative effort must involve the key decision makers from those interested organizations. The group must analyze benefits and risks of proceeding and weigh them against those of not moving forward with the project.

Two major factors influence whether there is sufficient interest in the project. The first stems from the topic being studied: Have a sufficient number of organizations committed to the effort so as to provide enough diversity from which to learn? That is, are the organizations sufficiently different that they have something to learn from one another on this topic? The second major factor is cost: Have enough organizations committed so that the project can be conducted cost effectively? The sponsoring organization may weigh these two issues when considering whether sufficient interest exists to proceed in a collaborative model.

The answer to "enough organizations" plays out differently in establishing collaboratives among stand-alone organizations. For example, a negative response to a collaborative being established within an existing structure generates three options: halt the effort, which defeats the improvement project; convince others within the existing group to join the collaborative, which may result in additional participants; or open participation up to organizations outside the existing body, an option that brings with it all the challenges inherent in establishing a benchmarking collaborative from freestanding organizations. When a collaborative formed from independent organizations responds to this question negatively, it has more limited options: halt the effort, which still defeats the purpose of the collaborative; broaden the net of potential participants and repeat exploring interest levels, which although it delays the effort allows it to continue to move forward; or reconsider the question of what constitutes "enough organizations."

Step 6: Identify and Educate Stakeholders

Once it has been shown that interest and commitment levels are sufficient for the project to proceed, the next step is to identify stakeholders in the collaborative so that appropriate communication and education campaigns can be designed. Communication serves to enhance stakeholder awareness and understanding of the study topic, including education on certain aspects of the study topic. These communication and education efforts become part of the work plan for the collaborative. (The specifics of education and training will be presented in chapter 8.)

Who the Stakeholders Are

In the benchmarking collaborative most stakeholders—beneficiaries of the successful execution of the project that results in improved organizational performance—come from participating organizations—senior leaders, middle managers, and members of the organizational benchmarking teams. Additional stakeholders include employees of the organizations involved and internal customers of the process under examination. Some stakeholders (for example vendors and suppliers) reside outside the organizations. Referring again to the workers' compensation example, the insurance broker is a stakeholder because the project outcome would have an impact on the business relationship between the health system and the broker.

Ultimate stakeholders are the patients or clients served by the health care facility. Even though they have vested interests in improvements that result from the benchmarking project, they may not be intimately involved in the effort. Therefore, they may require less communication from the team.

How Stakeholders Are Educated

Internal stakeholders need to understand overall project strategy, which involves communicating the intent of the project, rationale for selecting the project, and expected outcomes, as broadly defined. This "big picture" offers a contextual framework for stakeholders and promotes understanding of the reasons for involvement and participation.

Stakeholders also need to know what approach the collaborative will take to accomplish the project. If the context explains the "why" of the effort, the approach explains the "how." For some stakeholders, such as those not directly involved in conducting the study, an overview is adequate. That statement might be limited to delineating the underlying reasons for benchmarking collaboratively, a description of the organizations involved, and a summary of steps in the approach. Figure 5-4 summarizes the workers' compensation benchmarking project.

For those directly involved, more detailed communication and education is required so that unnecessary and repetitive activity does not take place, along with the frustration that accompanies it. Less frustration means acceptance of the project experience and higher likelihood of future participation.

Specific communication and education initiatives include training in benchmarking methodology and utilization of the tools and techniques of quality improvement. For organizations new to team-based improvement efforts, training in group dynamics may be required.

Figure 5-4. Benchmarking Project Summary Statement

- Project:

  Identify a model workers' compensation
  program for implementation within
  affiliated organizations

- Rationale:

  Current program costs
  Current facility costs
  Current occurrence rates

- Approach:

  Select project
  Establish collaborative
  PDSA within the collaborative
  PDSA with outside partners

Step 7: Create a Collaborative Project Charter

The benchmarking collaborative project charter describes the mission and purpose of the group. Charter components may include the following: definition of the group mission, a broad statement of what results members can expect from participation, requirements for participation, and ground rules for how the group will function. As a collaborative, the group must arrive at these elements through consensus.

The *mission statement*, which defines the purpose for which the collaborative was formed, describes the overall aim of the benchmarking effort. The *results* that members can expect represent the goals of the benchmarking project— goals which, at this stage, may at best be broadly defined. They may be refined later in the project.

If the group chooses to stipulate *conditions for participation*, it may include them in the charter. These conditions clarify who is eligible for participation. Again, using the workers' compensation project as an example, one condition for participation was that organizations had to come from states that permitted directed care of workers' compensation cases, a requirement that automatically eliminated certain organizations.

As with any team activity, establishing *ground rules* plays a critical role in predicting success. The collaborative may wish to include them in its charter to formalize how it will operate. (See figure 5-5.) (Chapter 8 explores the purpose of ground rules in more detail.)

Again, as with all other policy decisions, the collaborative must rely on group consensus in establishing a charter. Doing so builds teamship and furthers commitment to the charter. Figure 5-6 outlines the charter for the workers' compensation benchmarking collaborative.

While creating the project charter, the ultimate purpose of the benchmarking collaborative must remain at the forefront. That purpose is to support those organizations that want to bring about dramatic performance improvement of the selected project.

Figure 5-5. Examples of Ground Rules

- We start on time and end on time.
- We stay on track and help the team stay on track.
- We use data to drive our decisions.
- We speak clearly and succinctly.
- We work as a team to accomplish our goals.
- We keep the overall goal in mind at all times.
- Each member is responsible for our success.
- We practice active listening skills.
- We use clearly defined decision-making rules.
- We deal with conflict openly and honestly.
- We give everyone a chance to participate.
- We are sensitive to other team members' needs.

Figure 5-6. Workers' Compensation Charter Statement

- Project mission:
  Identify a model workers' compensation program for implementation within affiliated organizations

- Project goals:
  Reduce the current program costs
  Reduce the current facility costs
  Reduce the current occurrence rates

- Conditions for participation:
  Commitment to benchmarking methodology
  Commitment to team approach
  Commitment to implement results
  Geographic dispersion
  Facility type mix (acute or long-term care)
  Directed/nondirected care
  Mixed current experience
  Preferred TQM experience

Step 8: Adopt a Benchmarking Ethics Code

Before initiating the project and establishing a guidance team, the ethics and etiquette of benchmarking warrant some discussion. Because benchmarking activities are being conducted among a wide variety of industries, concerns over legal and ethical issues surrounding these activities have led leaders in the discipline to create a code of conduct. That code of conduct provides guidelines for practitioners, promotes professionalism within the practice, and enhances the effectiveness of benchmarking. The International Benchmarking Clearinghouse, a service of the American Productivity & Quality Center, and the Strategic Planning Institute Council on Benchmarking have adopted a common code of conduct.

This code of conduct rests on nine fundamental principles: legality, exchange, confidentiality, use, first-party contact, third-party contact, preparation, completion, and understanding and action. These principles (figure 5-7) form a set of standard behaviors that benchmarkers are expected to adhere to.

Figure 5-7. APQC Benchmarking Code of Conduct

Individuals agree for themselves and their company to abide by the following principles for benchmarking with other organizations.

1. Principle of *Legality*.

   1.1 If there is any potential question on the legality of an activity, don't do it.

   1.2 Avoid discussions or actions that could lead to or imply an interest in restraint of trade, market and/or customer allocation schemes, price fixing, dealing arrangements, bid rigging, or bribery. Don't discuss costs with competitors if costs are an element of pricing.

   1.3 Refrain from the acquisition of trade secrets from others by any means that could be interpreted as improper, including the breach or inducement of any duty to maintain secrecy. Do not disclose or use any trade secret that may have been obtained through improper means or that was disclosed by another in violation of a duty to maintain its secrecy or limit its use.

   1.4 Do not, as a consultant or client, extend one benchmarking study's findings to another company without first obtaining the permission of the parties of the first study.

2. Principle of *Exchange*.

   2.1 Be willing to provide the same type and level of information that you request from your benchmarking partner to your benchmarking partner.

   2.2 Communicate fully and early in the relationship to clarify expectations, avoid misunderstanding and establish mutual interest in the benchmarking exchange.

   2.3 Be honest and complete.

3. Principle of *Confidentiality*.

   3.1 Treat benchmarking interchange as confidential to the individuals and companies involved. Information must not be communicated outside the partnering organizations without the prior consent of the benchmarking partner who shared the information.

   3.2 A company's participation in a study is confidential and should not be communicated externally without their prior permission.

4. Principle of *Use*.

   4.1 Use information obtained through benchmarking only for purposes of formulating improvement of operations or processes within the companies participating in the benchmarking study.

   4.2 The use or communication of a benchmarking partner's name with the data obtained or observed practices requires the prior permission of that partner.

   4.3 Do not use benchmarking information or any information resulting from a bench-marking exchange, or benchmarking related networking as a means to market or sell.

   4.4 Contact lists or other contact information provided by the International Benchmarking Clearinghouse in any form may not be used for marketing in any way.

5. Principle of *First-Party Contact*.

   5.1 Initiate benchmarking contacts, whenever possible, through a benchmarking contact designated by the partner company.

   5.2 Respect the corporate culture of partner companies and work within mutually agreed procedures.

   5.3 Obtain mutual agreement with the designated benchmarking contact on any hand-off of communication or responsibility to other parties.

Figure 5-7. (Continued)

6. Principle of *Third-Party Contact*.

   6.1 Obtain an individual's permission before providing his/her name in response to a contact request.

   6.2 Avoid communicating a contact's name in an open forum without the contact's prior permission.

7. Principle of *Preparation*.

   7.1 Demonstrate commitment to the efficiency and effectiveness of benchmarking by being prepared prior to making an initial benchmarking contact.

   7.2 Make the most of your benchmarking partner's time by being fully prepared for each exchange.

   7.3 Help your benchmarking partners prepare by providing them with a questionnaire and agenda prior to benchmarking visits.

8. Principle of *Completion*.

   8.1 Follow through with each commitment made to your benchmarking partner in a timely manner.

   8.2 Complete each benchmarking study to the satisfaction of all benchmarking partners as mutually agreed.

9. Principle of *Understanding and Action*.

   9.1 Understand how your benchmarking partner would like to be treated.

   9.2 Treat your benchmarking partner in the way that your benchmarking partner would want to be treated.

   9.3 Understand how your benchmarking partners would like to have the information they provide handled and used, and handle and use it in that manner.

Reprinted, with permission, from The Healthcare Forum, copyright 1992.

An ethics code translates into practical behaviors for benchmarkers to follow during all phases of a project. The collaborative may adopt the code of conduct cited above or it may have one drafted by the legal council of one participating. Most of these behaviors follow the golden rule — treat others as you want to be treated. Benchmarkers are advised to go a step further, to the platinum rule — treat others as they want to be treated.[1] This extra step recognizes the inherent cultural differences in organizations, and effective benchmarkers understand and respect these differences.

Step 9: Initiate the Project and Select a Guidance Team

The collaborative is now ready to begin its project work. Individual organizations that begin the quality transformation need a quality council appointed to guide their initiative. Similarly, organizations that undertake a benchmarking project using a collaborative model need a group to guide and oversee their effort. This group can be made up from members of the collaborative or, if the collaborative is composed of more than 15 members, a subset of the group appointed to serve as the guidance team. As discussed earlier in this chapter, establishing a guidance team depends on the size and structure of the collaborative.

Whether through the guidance team or through the collaborative working as a group, two primary purposes drive the guidance team. The first is a task-oriented purpose, that is, to ensure success of the benchmarking project through accomplishing those steps necessary for completion. The second is a team-oriented purpose, to address needs and functional responsibilities of the team. The group must balance task and team purposes to achieve the desired results of the benchmarking project—improved organizational performance and healthier communities. Figure 5-8 presents a summary listing of these two purposes, which are further detailed in the following sections.

Task-Oriented Purposes

The task-driven purposes of the team include guiding the overall effort, planning the project, coordinating the efforts of participants, promoting active participation, communicating with participants and stakeholders, and educating participants. The primary task, however, is to lead the benchmarking effort by providing design and supervision to the project.

Developing a Plan

To plan effectively, the group must accomplish several subsidiary tasks, the most important of which is development of a detailed plan that lays out activities to be conducted by the guidance team and the benchmarking teams at participating organizations. This plan provides the road map the groups will follow on their journey through the benchmarking project. A work plan for the

Figure 5-8.   Task and Team Purposes of the Benchmarking Collaborative

Task-Oriented Purposes	Team-Oriented Purposes
Provide general guidance	Build shared vision and common purpose
Plan the project	Lay foundation for future collaboration
Coordinate specific efforts	Build group dynamics and team skills
Promote participation	
Communicate	
Develop and provide education	

workers' compensation project (figure 5-9) incorporates some steps performed by the staff of the sponsoring organization, as well as by the guidance team. It does not reflect all steps prescribed in the collaborative model but does demonstrate the level of detail, a possible format, and an overview of the work to be accomplished. Later chapters provide work plans specific to steps in the model.

The road map also provides participants with an understanding of the coordination required to bring the project to closure. This represents another purpose of the guidance team—to coordinate the benchmarking efforts within participating members of the benchmarking collaborative.

Promoting Participation and Communication with Stakeholders

The guidance team also helps promote active involvement in the benchmarking project among participating organizations. Although managers intuitively may find benchmarking appealing as a discipline, sustained participation often requires considerable selling of the approach and its inherent benefits. To maintain momentum and active participation, the guidance team must communicate with participating organizations on project purpose, progress, and results on a frequent and regular basis. To accomplish this, the team might use routine communication vehicles in the participating organizations—newsletters, meetings, letters, and memoranda.

Educating and Training Stakeholders

Preparing members of the group to embark on the project work requires development and provision of education and training on benchmarking tools and techniques. This training depends on the knowledge level of participants but might include a review of process analysis methods, measurement and statistics, and interviewing techniques. Benchmarking teams in participating organizations also may require some review of quality improvement skills such as basic process analysis and management techniques, as well as customer service training.

Training offers the collaborative an opportunity to tap the resources of participants. Because of the emphasis on continuous improvement in health care, most participants will likely already have the group dynamics and process management skills required by the team's effort. This gives the collaborative the chance to leverage existing resources for training in a cost-effective way.

If the collaborative requires outside help to meet its training needs, the group size can be an advantage in terms of gaining that help in a less costly manner. Further, the collaborative approach can incorporate a "train-the-trainer" model whereby a subgroup of the collaborative takes training in a specific topic and then trains the remainder of the collaborative. This approach could then be extended to the benchmarking teams of participating facilities. Chapter 8, "Management of the Benchmarking Team," addresses the training issue in more detail.

Figure 5-9. Workers' Compensation Work Plan

Date	Activity	Responsibility
January 1994	Concept presentation to management staff	RMR staff
	Identify potential participating organizations	RMR staff
	Select participating organizations	RMR staff
	Identify key decision makers	RMR staff
	Draft invitation to participate	RMR staff
February 1994	Send invitation to participate to facilities	RMR staff
	Initiate development of workers' compensation manual	RMR staff
	Initiate development of write-ups on American Disability Act & Family Medical Leave regulations impact on workers' compensation	HR staff
	Monthly management staff update	RMR staff
March 1994	Facilities agree to participate	Participating facilities
	Form guidance team	RMR staff and participating facilities
	Form facility benchmarking teams	Participating facilities
	Train facility benchmarking teams	Guidance team
	Complete data collection instrument	Guidance team
	Complete workers' compensation manual	RMR staff

Date	Activity	Responsibility
	Complete guidelines for facility benchmarking teams	Guidance team
	Complete write-ups on American Disability Act & Family Medical Leave Act	HR staff
	Monthly management staff update	RMR staff
April 1994	Send data collection instrument to participating facilities	Guidance team
	Participating facilities initiate data collection	Participating facilities
	Initiate search for external benchmarking partners and best practices	Guidance team
	Monthly management staff update	RMR staff
May 1994	Participating facilities continue data collection	Participating facilities
	Monthly management staff update	RMR staff
June 1994	Participating facilities return completed data collection instruments	Participating facilities
	Monthly management staff update	RMR staff
July 1994	Identify internal better practices	Guidance team
	Complete interview guide for external benchmarking partners	Guidance team
	Monthly management staff update	RMR staff
August 1994	Work with external benchmarking partners to identify best practices	Guidance team
	Monthly management staff update	RMR staff

(Continued on next page)

Figure 5-9. (Continued)

Date	Activity	Responsibility
September 1994	Identify lessons learned and implementable best practices	Guidance team
	HSC status report	Guidance team
	Monthly management staff update	RMR staff
October 1994	Initiate facility implementation	Participating facilities
	Initiate design of follow-up reporting and monitoring system	Guidance team
	Monthly management staff update	RMR staff
November 1994	Monthly management staff update	RMR staff
December 1994	Establish follow-up reporting and monitoring system	Guidance team
January 1995	HSC final report	Guidance team

Team-Oriented Purposes

Team-driven purposes include building a shared vision and common purpose, laying the foundation for future collaboration, and building group dynamics and team skills. The linchpin is building bridges for future collaborative efforts. These may entail additional benchmarking projects among the same participants, or they may go beyond the scope of a benchmarking project and branch into other areas, such as resource sharing or service delivery. Future collaboration rests on how well the current experience meets the functional and social (team) needs of participants.

Senge writes eloquently and articulately about the power of shared vision to coalesce a group.[2] The guidance team must define its vision for both the project and the group, beginning with a project charter that delineates the mission. If the sole focus of the group becomes completion of the study, then there is risk of losing future opportunities for learning and collaboration. This loss affects not only future "abstract" chances for cooperation, it directly compromises opportunities for follow-up learning from the current real project. Counterproductive experiences and relationships within the benchmarking collaborative decrease the likelihood for second- and third-level responses to inquiries on issues related to the benchmarking project. These lost opportunities decrease the effectiveness for learning and ultimately reduce the potential for continued breakthrough improvement.

The guidance team must build skills for collaboration and cooperation. Much like a quality improvement team within an individual organization, the guidance team may require specific training on group dynamics and team skills to function effectively. One purpose the group serves is to provide these skills to enhance its own performance and to increase the likelihood of successful accomplishment of the group tasks. The team builds these skills through working together in a way that establishes and reinforces trust.

Summary

The benchmarking collaborative provides a vehicle for organizations to learn from others facing similar challenges. Toward this end it builds relationships among participating organizations. This chapter focused on how collaboratives may be formed to reinforce relationships that focus attention on the project selected and on the cooperative effort. To be effective, the benchmarking collaborative must be small enough to function efficiently, yet large enough and diverse enough to provide ample opportunity for learning and comprehensive exploration of a topic. It brings together organizations that want to work cooperatively to seek breakthrough improvements in the process under study. Establishing the right collaborative in terms of size, group diversity, service mix, shared vision and purpose, task focus, and team focus all serve to distribute learning and cost savings optimally while promoting breakthrough improvements.

Putting These Ideas to Work

Objective

Identify and list the characteristics desired in members of your benchmarking collaborative.

Approach

Pose the following question for brainstorming: "What characteristics do organizations display that make them ideal members for our benchmarking collaborative?"

Answers to this question provide a foundation in three areas. First, desirable traits for benchmarking collaborative members will be identified. Second, this list leads to discussion of conditions for participation. Third, these two lists lead to discussion of ground rules for the benchmarking collaborative. Discuss the implications of these items and create the three following refined lists:

1. Desirable traits for members of your benchmarking collaborative
2. Possible conditions for participation
3. Potential ground rules

References

1. Mancusi, J. L. Cultural diversity: another view of the golden rule. *NewsCenter for Organizational Excellence*, 1991. (Newsletter published by the Center for Organizational Excellence, Fairfax Station, VA.)

2. Senge, P. *The Fifth Discipline*. New York City: Doubleday/Currency, 1990, pp. 205–32.

Phase 3: Conduct Internal Study

Introduction

With the benchmarking project selected and the collaborative formed, the stage is set for benchmarking within the collaborative, that is, conducting an internal study. Building on the project charter, the collaborative first plans and conducts the study among its members, using an adaptation of Shewhart's Plan-Do-Study-Act cycle as shown in figure 6-1.

This chapter describes each phase of the model. The *Plan* component involves development of the overall blueprint for action, a timetable for executing each activity related to the project, and a general goal for improvement. Benchmarking teams in participating organizations develop internal project plans. The *Do* phase is spent describing and analyzing the current process in each organization so that each benchmarking team understands its own work process(es). The *Study* segment involves searching for best practices within the collaborative. Members compile and analyze the results and identify any best practices disclosed by the study. The *Act* phase is characterized by implementation of best practices found in the collaborative. Once this occurs, benchmarking teams implement, evaluate, and monitor improvements in their organizations.

Plan

Planning for the internal phase of the benchmarking study occurs at two levels. The first is at the level of the collaborative, and the second is at the organizational level.

Collaborative Plan

The collaborative or its guidance team must ensure that the project stays focused on the topic selected and on related strategic improvements. At this level, the study plan establishes the boundaries of the process to be improved, as represented by the beginning and ending steps of a macro (high-level) flowchart. The project

Figure 6-1. Internal Plan-Do-Study-Act Cycle

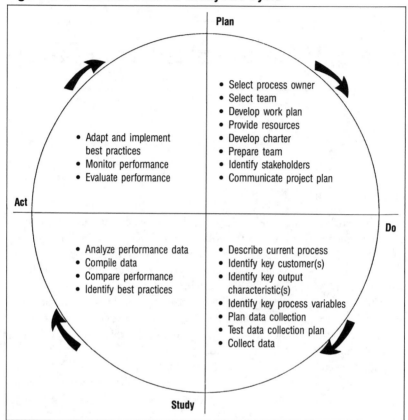

plan facilitates coordination among participants in the collaborative and provides a framework to guide the project within each member organization. The collaborative work plan outlines major activities and target dates and serves as a road map to keep the project moving efficiently toward completion.

Figure 6-2 shows the plan developed by the guidance team for the workers' compensation study referred to in chapters 2 and 3. Each phase of the collaborative benchmarking model is included, along with major steps to be completed in each phase following project selection.

Organizational Plan

Planning for the internal phase of benchmarking continues in each participating organization, as its quality council (or administrative team) selects the process owner and a team and develops the study plan. Other activities include providing resources, developing a charter, preparing the team, identifying stakeholders, and communicating with all involved parties.

Figure 6-2. Collaborative Plan: Workers' Compensation Study Timetable

Select project	December 1993–January 1994
Form collaborative	February–March 1994
• Determine project goals • Determine data collection requirements for collaborative • Charter organizational benchmarking teams • Train teams	
Conduct internal study	*March–July 1994*
• Organizational benchmarking teams plan and complete study *• Teams report results* *• Collaborative compiles results* *• Teams search for internal best practices* *• Teams implement best practices* *• Collaborative decides on external study*	
Conduct external study	August–September 1994
• Develop detailed plan • Identify partners • Conduct study • Identify best practices	
Implement best practices	October 1994
• Benchmarking teams adapt and implement • Monitor results and report to collaborative	

Select the Process Owner

On the organizational level, the first planning step is to identify the process owner—that individual who is or *could be* responsible for most operational components of the cross-functional process to be studied. The owner provides leadership and support for conducting the study and for implementation of the resulting improvements. Identification of process ownership is especially important because complex, cross-functional processes have typically been "unmanaged." Naturally, it is often difficult to identify who owns such processes.

The quality council or senior management team looks for the following characteristics in the process owner/benchmarking team leader:

- Credibility
- Innovativeness
- CQI awareness
- Benchmarking awareness
- CQI and benchmarking advocacy
- Availability (15–20 percent of time)

If the quality council and benchmarking team perceive the process owner as credible and innovative, this will significantly influence their acceptance of project outcomes and the extent to which senior managers drive implementation of improvements. Comprehension of the organization's CQI and benchmarking efforts can, of course, be learned by the owner. Although support of the CQI and benchmarking efforts is more difficult to ensure, this characteristic can be developed and reinforced by senior management. The team leader should be able to dedicate 15 to 20 percent of his or her time to the project.

If a process owner cannot be found who sufficiently embodies these characteristics, the quality council may identify a sponsor from its own ranks to support the process owner. Councils often assign senior executives to act as sponsors or champions for benchmarking projects in order to demonstrate support and the priority placed on breakthrough improvement. If 15–20 percent of the process owner's time cannot be made available to lead the study, the council may identify a co-leader or an alternate leader, so long as the process owner is closely involved in the project.

For example, organizations in the workers' compensation study selected human resources and risk management professionals as process owners for their benchmarking teams. Not only were they intimately involved with the process of workers' compensation, these managers had been involved in the organizations' CQI efforts and had experience as members or leaders of improvement teams.

Select the Team

The process owner (with the sponsor or quality council) selects the benchmarking team to conduct the project within each participating organization. By definition, benchmarking, like most improvement efforts, is a team activity. A team is necessary for several reasons. Understanding a complex process requires the combined expertise of those who work in the process. On a practical level, project demands dictate sharing the work load, and a team effort generates cross-departmental support for the improvements to be made as a result of that project.

Because benchmarking involves the study of processes that operate across functional lines, teams should be cross-functional and interdepartmental in their makeup. These teams also should be *ad hoc in nature*, that is, organized for the duration of the project, and then generally disbanded after implementation of improvements.

Along with the process owner/team leader, the benchmarking team is made up of 3 to 10 people who have some knowledge of the process to be improved. To keep the team at a manageable size, it is recommended that only those necessary to understand the process from the first to the last step be included as standing members.

In the workers' compensation project, organizational benchmarking teams consisted of managers and professionals with knowledge of the workers' compensation process. These included senior operations executives; representatives from finance, human resources, risk management, and employee health; and quality management professionals. Actual team sizes varied among participants, ranging anywhere from four to eight.

The benchmarking team is also likely to be supported by one or more internal or external professionals trained in benchmarking methods and tools. This is especially true in organizations without previous benchmarking experience. In the workers' compensation project, quality professionals served as team facilitator/advisers. Another support role, as mentioned earlier, is that of the project sponsor. Each of these roles and the preparation and management of the benchmarking team are addressed in chapter 8.

Develop a Work Plan

The benchmarking project sponsor (or quality council), the team leader, and the facilitator/adviser or benchmarking specialist jointly develop a work plan (project plan) for the project. The work plan or road map identifies activities and target completion dates for the project and serves as a reference point for the project team. (See figure 6-3.) Scope of the project is a primary factor in developing a timetable. Generally, internal collaborative projects will require four to six months to complete. The time line is coordinated with that of the plan established by the collaborative guidance team. The activities of the internal benchmarking cycle identified in chapter 3 and those described in this chapter serve as an excellent model for what to include in the plan.

The work plan provides for team progress reports to the quality council and guidance team at regular intervals, not only to support the team but to promote learning and to keep attention focused on this strategically important activity.

Consultation with the guidance team and other members of the collaborative ensures that project plans for the internal study are coordinated. It also facilitates a consistent approach among the benchmarking teams. A model plan provided by the guidance team facilitates project execution within the organization. An alternative is for members of the collaborative to provide plans to the guidance team, which evaluates them for consistency.

Provide Resources

Senior management or the quality council authorizes budget and time allocations for the benchmarking project. For the organizational phase of the study, the budget will consist primarily of release time for project work and, if used, the fees and expenses of external experts. Costs of computer software and supplies (such as flipcharts, markers, stationery, and the like) also may be included. These resource oversight activities provide the team with the means needed to execute the project while guiding the use of scarce resources. Just as important, they demonstrate explicit organizational support for the project, both to

Figure 6-3. Organizational Plan for Internal Benchmarking Cycle: Workers' Compensation Study

March	April	May	June	July
Plan • Select team • Develop work plan • Provide resources • Develop team charter • Prepare team • Identify stakeholders • Communicate project to stakeholders	**Do** • Describe current process • Identify key customers • Identify KOC(s) • Identify KPV(s) • Plan data collection • Report to council	• Test data collection plan • Collect data	**Study** • Analyze data • Report to council • Compile results • Compare performance • Identify best practices	**Act** • Implement best practices • Monitor performance • Evaluate results • Report

Key: KOC = Key output characteristic
      KPV = Key process variable

management and to the benchmarking team, thus ensuring the priority of the project in relation to other organizational activities. Careful provision and utilization of resources also raise expectations of the team, the council, and management for successful project completion.

Develop the Project Charter

The quality council summarizes the project planning in a team project charter, a document that includes a statement of the mission or benchmarking opportunity, composition of the project team, the work plan, and the budget. As it develops this charter, the council uses the larger collaborative charter (described in chapter 5) as a guide for planning the organizational study.

Prepare the Team

Team orientation is conducted by the project sponsor and the team leader. The orientation meeting includes an introduction to each element of the charter as well as, perhaps, a team-building activity (for example, an ice-breaker segment during which members introduce themselves and give new information like favorite hobbies or a fantasy vacation spot). Next, if members have never been involved in a previous study, the team is trained in benchmarking methodology. This might involve an overview of the collaborative approach and the steps involved, presented by the facilitator/adviser or a consultant. Specific tools used at each step are introduced as they are needed by the team. This "just-in-time" training typically is provided by the facilitator/adviser. A more detailed description of training content, as well as of methods for developing and managing the benchmarking team, is offered in chapter 8.

Identify Stakeholders

Project stakeholders (as distinguished from collaborative stakeholders discussed in chapter 5) are those who receive any output of the process selected for the benchmarking project, those who have investment in project outcomes, and those who may benefit from understanding the results of the project. In the workers' compensation study, staff members who have filed claims and their managers were stakeholders who received outputs of the process. Physicians, the insurance broker, and central office risk managers also were affected directly. Chief executive officers and chief financial officers in each participating organization also had an investment in the financial impact of the study, as did regional vice-presidents and the insurance committee of the board. Quality advisers and managers who had never dealt with a workers' compensation claim were also potential beneficiaries of the project.

The quality council and the team identify stakeholders to keep the benchmarking team focused on producing usable outcomes from the project, define important communication targets, and increase the likelihood of successfully implementing improvements. To identify stakeholders, the council and the team draw on their knowledge of the organization, customers and suppliers, and of the process being benchmarked. Typically this involves a simple brainstorming exercise, perhaps followed by a multivote to determine priority stakeholders.

Communicate with Stakeholders

As the benchmarking project is launched, senior management informs the stakeholders of the effort. This calls attention to the importance of the project and of breakthrough improvement, builds support for the team and the project, and enhances the credibility of those who make up the benchmarking team. Generally this communication occurs through regular channels such as management meetings and house organs, with special attention to reaching key stakeholders outside the organization.

The guidance team for the workers' compensation project initially informed stakeholders of the study, provided copies of the work plan, and reported progress at regular intervals. They used existing communication methods such as newsletters and a special report at the conclusion of the project.

The Planning Role of the Benchmarking Team

The benchmarking team also plays a role in planning the project. As one of its first activities, the team reviews the stakeholders or customers of the project results and plans for how it will communicate during the course of the study. Common approaches include management meetings and special vehicles like team storyboards.

The team also reviews the work plan and develops it in further detail as necessary to guide the project. For example, the workers' compensation benchmarking teams developed more specific steps and timetables within each phase of the road map provided by their quality councils. This planning included detailed agendas for each team meeting and steps and time frames for collecting data on process performance.

Do

The Do phase of a collaborative benchmarking project cycle closely parallels the work of a quality improvement team. Like any quality improvement team, the benchmarking team depends on a thorough understanding of the existing process and its performance. This is necessary for several reasons:

- To ensure that customer requirements are clearly identified
- To document how the process presently operates
- To quantify the performance of the process
- To facilitate later adaptation of benchmark practices

During this phase of benchmarking the team employs basic quality improvement tools: flowcharting; cause-effect analysis; data collection; and the graphic tools of descriptive statistics, such as run charts or Pareto analysis. Specific activities of the Do phase, from describing the current process to collecting data for analysis, are explained in the subsections that follow.

Describe the Current Process

The team begins its work by flowcharting the steps of the current process. The first flowchart will be a high-level identification of major steps in the process, as illustrated in figure 6-4, from the workers' compensation study.

Figure 6-4. Workers' Compensation Macro Process

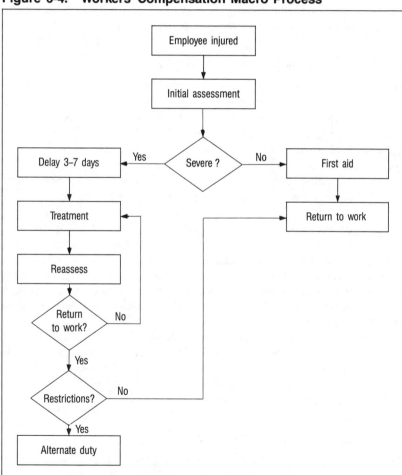

Next the team completes a detailed flowchart to get a closer look at how the process, or its critical components, currently operates. Figure 6-5 details the flow of the patient registration process in one of the hospitals in the admitting study undertaken by the American Productivity & Quality Center and The Healthcare Forum.[1]

Based on its knowledge of the process, the team analyzes the flowcharts to identify rework, redundancy, nonvalue-added steps, delays, waste, or errorproneness. The team later uses this analysis to identify key process variables and to plan for data collection. Although not its primary purpose, the flowchart enables the team to implement obvious, easy improvements in the process. Flowcharting the process also calls attention to variation in how it is operated, for example, from shift to shift or employee to employee. When one process is carried out in multiple ways without good reason, the team minimizes undue variation by adopting a common process for the duration of the study. Later, teams will examine the flowcharts of the same process from other organizations in the collaborative or from an external partner.

Identify Key Customer(s) and Requirements

The benchmarking team confirms or, if necessary, identifies the key customer(s) of the process. This ensures that the benchmarking project is focused on those stakeholders who depend on how the process performs. Although key customer(s) usually will be apparent, some application of the 80–20 rule may be useful in their selection; that is, concentrate on the customers most affected by the process being examined. In the workers' compensation study, for example, teams identified key customers as employees, insurance claims processors, and participating organizations, because the process has the greatest impact on these three groups.

If the team has sufficient current knowledge of key customer(s), it simply confirms customer requirements. If, however, these requirements are unknown or undocumented, or if knowledge about the customer is dated, the team must identify and document current customer needs of the process. In the workers' compensation study, teams determined that employees wanted a claims process that was simple and respectful of claimants. Employers naturally required a return to work as soon as appropriate; CEOs and CFOs needed a process that would save their organizations unnecessary expense.

Popular methods for learning about customer requirements include focus groups, interviews, and surveys. Limited knowledge of the customer may be derived from complaints, satisfaction surveys, or comment cards, although such information is less useful than more direct inquiry. (A number of excellent references offer in-depth discussion of these and other methods.[2-5])

Identify Key Output Characteristic(s)

The team establishes the *key output characteristic(s)* (KOC) of the process based on its knowledge of key customer requirements. The KOC is the operational, measurable definition of a customer requirement. For example, if the customer

Figure 6-5. Benchmarking the Inpatient Admitting Process

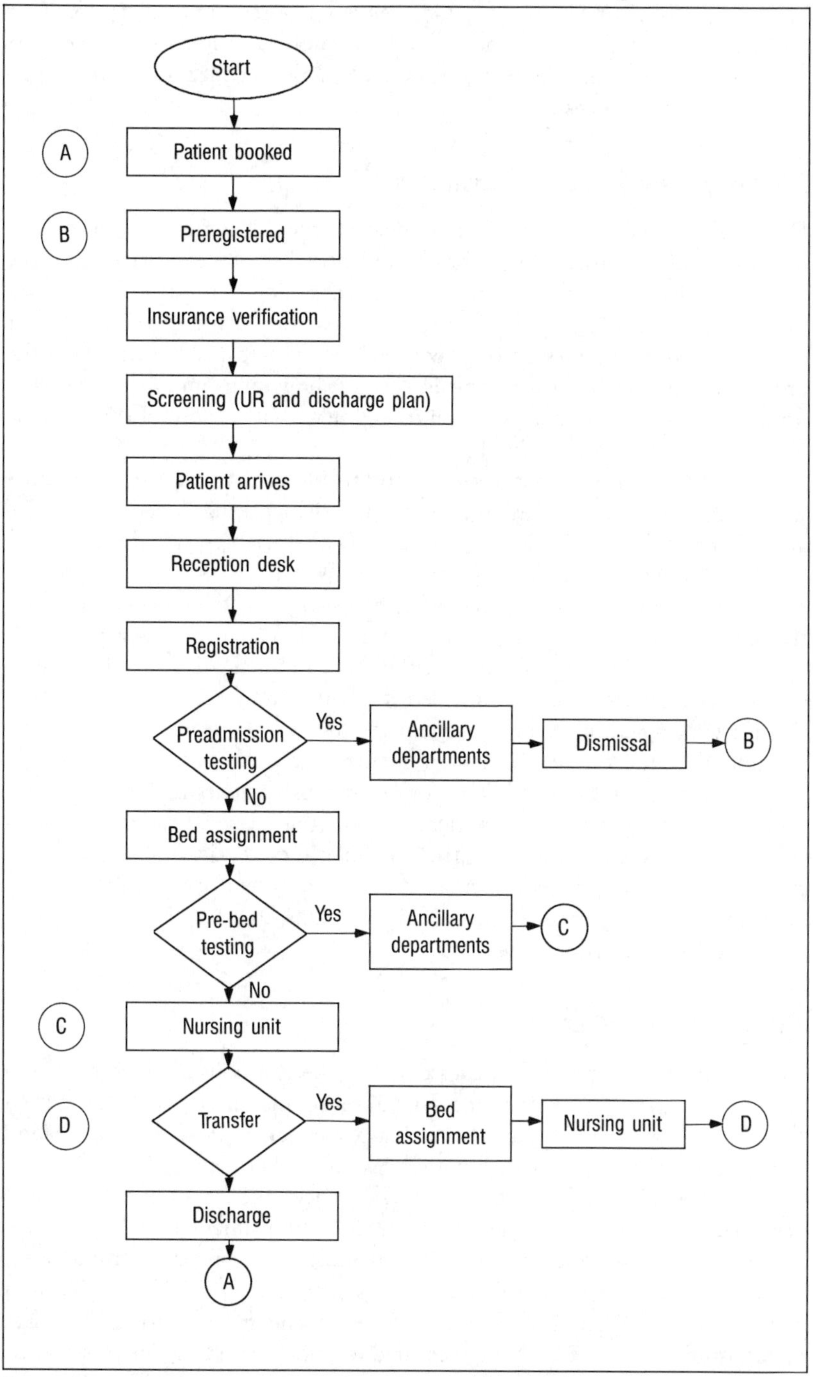

Reprinted, with permission, from *The Healthcare Forum,* copyright 1992.

requires an accurate patient bill, the KOC might be the number of errors found in patient bills. If timeliness of service delivery is a requirement, the KOC is based on the process cycle time, that is, turnaround time or wait time. The team must identify and define the KOC to be able to collect data on the performance of the process.

Identify Key Process Variables

Defining the KOC requires knowledge of the customer's requirements. Knowledge of the process helps the team identify key process variables—those "causes" or elements within the process that determine or influence how it performs. The workers' compensation teams knew that at a macro level, senior executives required a process that reduced cost. The teams' knowledge of the process told them that one variable in cost was how long employees were away from work. At a more detailed level, they knew that a cause of this variable was the employee's fitness level.

Using its knowledge of the process and the flowchart, the team determines what variables operate in the process. Generally speaking, a cause-effect diagram is the tool of choice to identify key process variables, but the team may use the affinity tool or a tree diagram instead. Whichever method is employed, the result is a graphic description of what happens inside the process to produce the outcome for the customer. (Chapter 3 includes a chart that suggests which tools are most appropriate for each step of the benchmarking study. References on process analysis tools are provided in chapter 8.)

Drawing again on its knowledge of the process, the team agrees on those variables thought to have the most influence on the key outcome characteristic. These variables are candidates for *key process variables* (KPVs), those few elements in the process that most affect how the process performs.

During this step of the study, the team may also identify "process enablers," practices or support processes that facilitate the performance of the process they are studying. Examples might be training programs, the availability of technology, or organizational culture.

Plan Data Collection

Collecting and analyzing data is essential to the team's understanding of the current process and its performance. In addition, this activity enables the team to compare process performance with that of partners in the collaborative (and later with that of external benchmarking partners). Ultimately, data inform the collaborative's identification of benchmark practices, the extent of improvement achieved, and the monitoring of new practices implemented.

The team plans for data collection to measure the process performance—both its outcome and the variables at work within the process. Identification of KOC(s) and selection of KPV candidates lay the groundwork for the data collection plan, in that both are measured to understand how the process performs and what causes it to vary.

Although collecting data need not be complicated or time consuming, it must be carefully planned. The benchmarking team can follow a step-by-step methodology to prevent rework and ensure that the data provide the information needed. An excellent set of questions to guide data collection planning has been developed by Paul Plsek.[6] These seven questions, in slightly modified form, are discussed below and incorporated in the matrix shown in figure 6-6.

What Question(s) Do We Need to Answer?

In general terms, the team needs to answer two basic questions: "How is the process currently performing (in terms of KOC)?" and "What are the most frequently occurring KPVs?" For example, in the workers' compensation project, a KOC for employers is number of employee days away from work. Teams then asked what were the most frequently occurring KPVs affecting employee days away from work. It is essential that all teams in the collaborative use the same questions to ensure that a common framework is used to guide data collection.

What Data Analysis Tools Will Help Us Answer These Questions?

The team anticipates what tools it will likely use in analyzing the data collected. The tools selected direct the team to the type of data needed and how much is to be collected. The tools of descriptive statistics usually serve the benchmarking process well: the run chart displays process performance over time; the Pareto diagram points to the "vital few" variables that affect the performance of the process. These tools are sometimes complemented by the histogram, which shows patterns in the distribution of the data; a control chart, where a more precise understanding of variation is required; and/or a scatter diagram, which examines the relationship between a variable and the KOC or between two variables.

What Type of Data Will Enable Us to Use the Tool(s) and Will Provide the Information We Need?

If, for example, a team expects to use a run chart, it will plan to collect either count (attribute) or measurement (variable) data, depending on how the KOC is defined. For example:

If the KOC is:	The type of data will be:
Number of errors in patient bills	Counts (a tally of number of errors)
Elapsed time for lab results	Measurement (timing the process and segments of it)
Cost of procedure	Measurement (computing cost)
Frequency of postsurgical infection	Counts (counting the number of infections)

Figure 6-6. Data Collection Planning Matrix

What do we need to know?	Analysis tool(s)	Type(s) of data	Data collection tool(s)	Sources		When		Responsibility
				Where	Who	Pilot	Actual	

Reprinted, with permission, from VHA Tri-State.

Do the Data Exist? At What Steps in the Process Can We Gather Them?

Even though existing data are rarely comprehensive enough or specific enough to describe process performance and variable frequency, the team first determines whether such data are available. If so, the team reviews it to be sure it meets the requirements of the data collection plan before proceeding with data analysis. Typically, the data collection plan must be completed, because most teams must collect current data. The flowchart serves as a helpful guide to identify data collection points within the process. It also highlights sources of data already available in the process, such as existing databases. Examples in health care include patient records and data collected for quality assurance purposes.

Who in the Process Can Assist Us in Collecting Data?

Whenever possible, members of the benchmarking team collect the data, or at least provide oversight for the effort. This provides team members with first-hand knowledge of the data while also ensuring that data are collected consistently by involving as few people as possible. When the team itself cannot collect data, it engages the minimum necessary number of associates who work in the process. In addition to keeping data collection simple, this strategy builds ownership for later improvements among those who operate the process. As a last resort, carefully trained and supervised external data collectors (such as graduate students) may be utilized.

How Can We Collect Data As Simply and Efficiently As Possible?

The "keep it simple" principle applies to data collection just as it does to other activity, especially where time and human resources are limited. The benchmarking team applies three criteria in planning for the collection of data: minimum effort, minimum time, and minimum chance of error or bias. Data collection forms and the steps followed in recording the data are designed as simply as possible in order to ensure that data collectors can go about their work easily, quickly, and with minimal chance of error.

What Additional Data or Information Do We Need to Help Us Understand the Process?

The team tries to anticipate what other useful data or information to gather at the same time process data are collected. This additional information usually falls into two categories: strata for data analysis and sources of special cause variation. For example, if the process being studied involves multiple shifts, operators, or equipment, the team will identify these strata for later analysis. If performance of the process is affected by external variables (such as the negative impact of a multicar accident on emergency room wait times or the positive effect of a process enabler), notes may be taken on special circumstances that might turn out to be special causes operating outside the process.

Of special interest to benchmarking teams is the identification of *process enablers*, those activities that support a breakthrough process or may make it easier to implement best practices.[7] For example, the on-line patient information system used by Intermountain Health Care has been an important enabler of their breakthrough improvement in selected clinical processes. Other examples might be training, supplier relations, or communication processes. When teams later adapt and implement best practices, they pay particular attention to these enablers, because they may be critical covariables with best practices. When an enabler is not present in its own organization or process, the team may want to introduce the enabler concurrently with incorporating the best practice. As a last step in planning, the team confirms the assignment of responsibility for various activities in the data collection plan.

Test the Data Collection Plan

Before proceeding with collecting data, the team tests the data collection plan by using the PDSA cycle. This testing process is explained in the following subsections.

Plan

Data collection planning activities culminate in a test of the plan. The plan is reviewed, with emphasis on what data will be gathered, the method to be used, and the timetable for the effort. Data collectors are trained and oriented as necessary, and informed of sources of assistance for questions or problems. If data are collected by people outside the benchmarking team, explanation of how the data will be used is a very important part of orientation. Explaining data application serves two purposes: It relieves any misgivings among data collectors about the purpose of the study, thus minimizing defensiveness and, therefore, potential bias. At the same time, it increases ownership of future improvements.

Do

The team uses the plan to collect actual data for a designated period. Testing time will vary, depending on the cycle time for the process under study. If the cycle time involves only minutes, testing time might last a few hours. If the process takes a few hours, the test might run a day or two. If the cycle time lasts from several hours to one day, a week's test time might be needed.

Study

The process itself is evaluated, along with the data already collected. Improvements to the data collection process, if any, are suggested. Test data are examined for obvious bias, error, or unexpected data. The data collection process and forms are also evaluated, using feedback from data collectors and/or team members. The team identifies lessons learned or improvements to be made before data collection gets under way.

Act

Necessary changes are made before data collection begins formally, including any improvements identified during the Study phase. If major changes are indicated, the PDSA test cycle may be repeated.

Collect Data

Having tested its plan, the benchmarking team collects data on the process selected for benchmarking. Team members continue to monitor the data collection process, especially as it begins, to ensure that bias, error, and problems are minimized. This is done by examining the data collected to be sure it shows variation and that the range of variation is generally what the team expects from the process. The team proceeds to gather and compile the data in preparation for analysis.

Study

During the Study phase each benchmarking team analyzes performance of the process in its organization to fully understand how the process operated in the way it did and why. Then the collaborative guidance team compiles results from participating organizations and compares performance data. The purpose is to determine whether best practices exist within the collaborative.

Analyze Performance Data: Benchmarking Teams

As is true with data collected for any quality improvement effort, the team first analyzes process performance data to ensure that the process is stable. In other words, data are examined for special cause variation by applying various tests for the presence of runs, trends, or repeat patterns.[8,9] This is accomplished with either a run chart or, where precision or sensitivity require it, a control chart. *Beneficial special causes,* such as process enablers or individual practices that produce exceptional results (the surgeon, for example, whose patients recover faster because she consistently makes a slightly smaller incision), are noted as possible improvements for later implementation. *Undesirable special causes* are studied and, if outside the control of the process owners and operators (for instance, equipment downtime resulting from a power outage), the related data points are noted and eliminated from further consideration. If the special cause can be controlled, the team takes action to do so. For instance, if data on elapsed time to admit patients indicate a special cause related to availability of transport equipment, the team works with the appropriate department on ways to ensure that equipment is accessed more easily.

Once the team is satisfied that the process is stable, the data collected on process variables are analyzed. Typically, Pareto analysis is used to identify the critical few variables, perhaps a single KPV. If KPVs are apparent in the Pareto diagram, the team has evidence of what influences performance of the process. (See figure 6-7.)

Figure 6-7   Pareto Diagram: Reasons for O₂ Desaturation

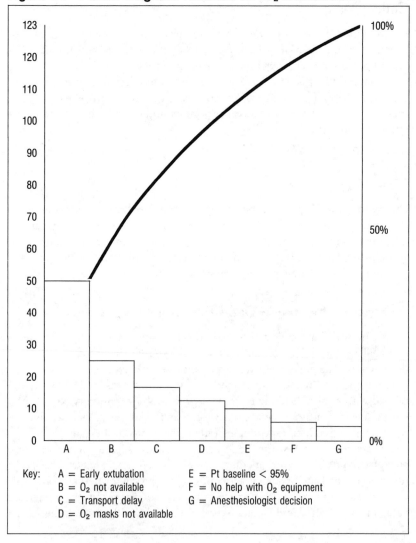

Key: A = Early extubation   E = Pt baseline < 95%
        B = O₂ not available   F = No help with O₂ equipment
        C = Transport delay   G = Anesthesiologist decision
        D = O₂ masks not available

In many cases, the relationship between the KPV(s) and the KOC will be obvious, based on data analysis and the team's understanding of the process. When this is not the case, or when greater precision is necessary—as in what effect a specific medication shows in a patient treatment process—further analysis of the relationship may be required. The scatter diagram may be used here. Figure 6-8, for example, illustrates the relationship between entry-to-fill time and total turnaround time in filling pharmacy orders.

The benchmarking team examines its findings carefully for the presence of process enablers that support performance of the process. Identifying and reporting process enablers to the collaborative guidance team is of special importance, particularly in relation to potential best practices. The on-line patient information system of Intermountain Health Care, mentioned earlier in this chapter, is an excellent illustration of a process enabler for many clinical care processes.

Figure 6-9 summarizes the path the team follows in studying an internal process. On the outcomes side, the customer of the process is identified, requirements are determined, and a measurable indicator of process performance is

Figure 6-8. Scatter Diagram: Time Relationship in Filling Pharmacy Orders

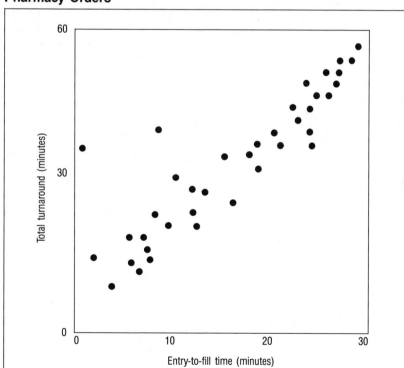

Figure 6-9. Understanding Process Performance

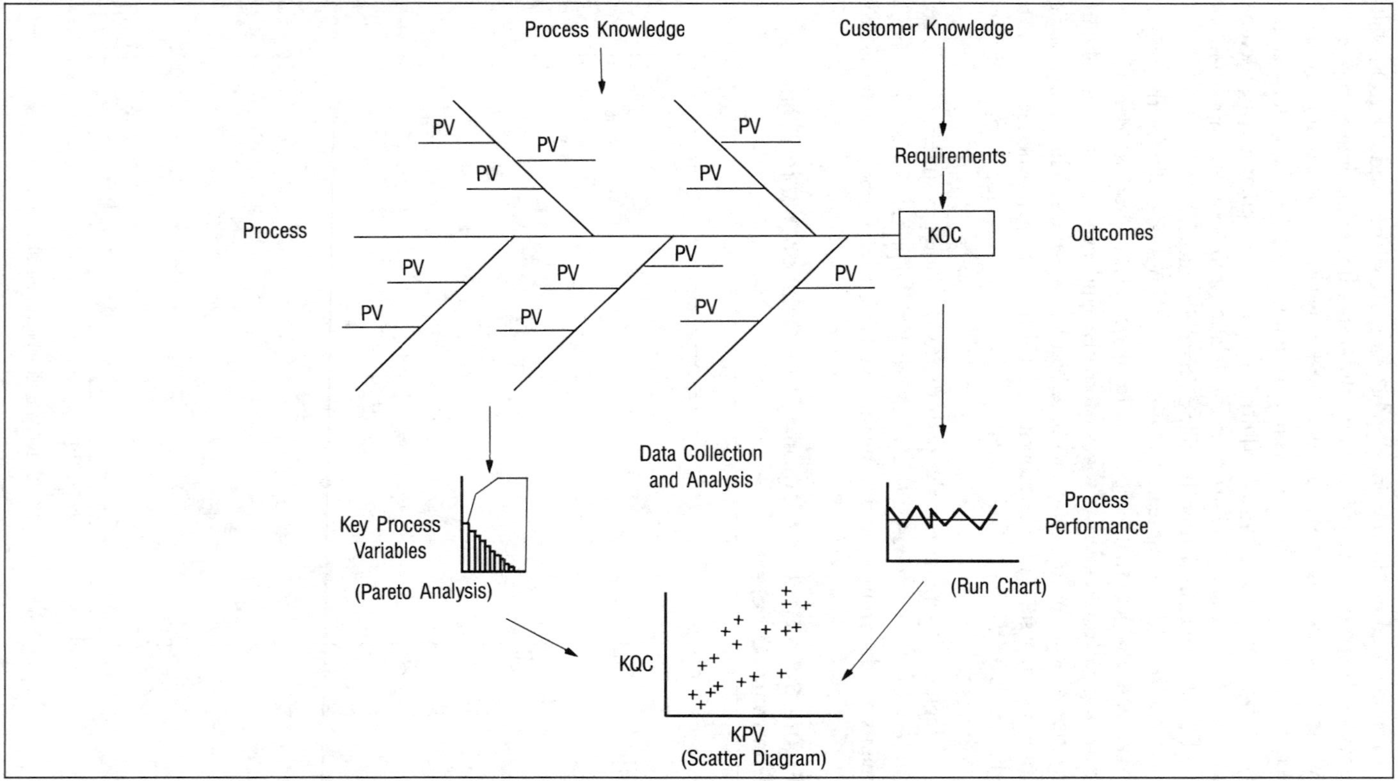

defined. The output of the process is commonly displayed on a run chart (or a control chart). On the process side, the team pools its expertise in how the work is done to identify process variables (PV on the diagram) that affect process output. These are recorded as the "bones" of the cause-effect diagram. Data are collected on frequency of variables the team hypothesizes to have most influence on how the process performs. These data are usually displayed on a Pareto chart, which identifies the "critical few" variables—the KPVs.

Compile Data: Guidance Team

Benchmarking teams report their findings to the guidance team, which compiles the summary data, stratified by organizations in the collaborative. At a minimum, these results include data on process performance and on key variables affecting that performance. An example of a summary of performance results from the SunHealth emergency services study is shown in figure 6-10.[10]

Figure 6-11 displays the same SunHealth performance data on a spider diagram, also known as a radar chart, which provides a more graphic representation of elapsed time for hospital 4, the organization with shortest time in the ER. Such use of descriptive statistics facilitates the data-driven identification of best practices.

Compare Performance and Identify Best Practices: Guidance Team

The guidance team now analyzes the data for potential best practices among members of the collaborative. First the team compares KOC performance, checking

Figure 6-10.   Emergency Services Summary of Key Data: July 8, 1991–July 15, 1991 (time reported in minutes)

	Hospitals 1–10									
Elapsed time from:	1	2	3	4	5	6	7	8	9	10
Patient enters department to first ES contact	4	8.5	8.5	.5	n/a	1.5	9	4	.5	3
Patient enters department to patient enters room	28	67	14.5	15.5	20.5	26	53	28.5	19.5	20.5
Patient enters department to doctor begins treatment	41	84	48	29	51.5	55.5	81.5	64	38	34.5
Patient enters room to doctor begins treatment	15.5	23	36	14.5	31	31	34.5	36	18.5	14.5

Reprinted, with permission, from SunHealth.

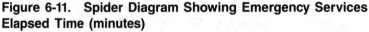

Figure 6-11. Spider Diagram Showing Emergency Services Elapsed Time (minutes)

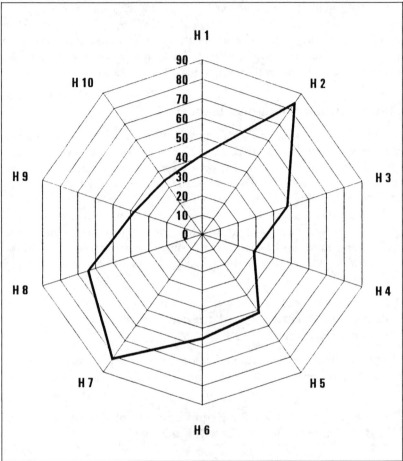

for breakthrough outcomes. If these are found, the guidance team refines the general improvement goal by establishing a realistic numerical target. In other words, the preliminary goal, which may be very broadly based on customer requirements, is now made more precise because the study data define the gap between the benchmark performance and all others. Data on performance variables are examined to determine any unique KPVs or process enablers that result in the benchmark performance. Key process variables with a strong, positive correlation with breakthrough results will often be reliable evidence of a best practice.

Act

During the Act phase of the internal study, best practices, if any, are implemented within the collaborative. Each benchmarking team adapts the benchmark practices and any related enablers and develops a plan for incorporating them into its own process. This includes collecting of data to measure performance against the goal.

Implement Best Practices

If best practices are found within the collaborative, the guidance team reports these to member organizations of the collaborative. Benchmarking teams identify the gaps between the performance of their own process and that of the benchmark process. In the SunHealth study, for example, hospital 7 might compare its performance with that of hospital 4, which would point out a gap of more than two hours. Next, using the report of the guidance team, the benchmarking team would study the practices of hospital 4. The team would then develop plans to adapt and implement the key variables and practice enablers identified in the guidance team analysis.

Whether the improvement plan involves incorporating benchmark practices into an existing process, redesign of the process, or development of a new process, the PDSA cycle is used: *Plan* the improvement systematically—first as a pilot—including steps to be taken, barriers to be overcome, support required, and data to be collected. *Do* the pilot run of the process—a limited scale or limited time, perhaps a simulation—including actual data collection. *Study* the results to determine whether target performance was achieved and to identify lessons learned to ensure later success. *Act* on the lessons learned as the process is standardized as the organization's new way of doing the work.

Monitor and Evaluate Performance

Benchmarking teams build into their implementation plans strategies for ongoing monitoring of performance to ensure that gains are held and also to facilitate continued improvement. Continued monitoring might take the form of a run chart or control chart of the KOC, which might be kept by the process owner or an appropriate member of the team. In either case, monitoring process performance occurs during operation of the process. As with any critical process, a trend in performance away from the goal signals the need to reexamine the process. This evaluation might lead to forming an improvement team or to reconvening the benchmarking team.

If the target performance is not achieved anywhere in the collaborative as a result of the internal benchmarking study, the guidance team and the collaborative decide whether to continue the study with external partners, the subject of chapter 7.

Summary

This chapter described the journey taken by the collaborative through the first internal cycle of benchmarking. After selecting a topic and establishing the collaborative, a project plan is developed to coordinate the study of the work process in each member organization. The goal is to develop a thorough understanding of process operations and process outcomes, including critical variables that affect performance. The collaborative then studies the results, in search of best practices among its members. If best practices are found, they are implemented in each organization and results are monitored to determine whether the necessary level of performance has been reached or exceeded. If no best practices are identified in the collaborative, or if sufficient performance improvement is not achieved, the collaborative begins the external cycle of benchmarking.

The internal benchmarking study closely resembles the work of a quality improvement team, in that organizational benchmarking teams use process analysis tools to map how the work is done, measure process performance, and identify key variables operating the process. The framework for the entire study is the Shewhart cycle: Plan-Do-Study-Act. Thus the internal cycle of benchmarking builds on the CQI experiences of health care organizations in terms of methods and tools.

Putting These Ideas to Work

Objective

Explore your understanding of a key process or subprocess in your organization.

Approach

1. Recall the process you selected in chapter 4.
2. Evaluate your understanding of that process in terms of the guidelines presented in this chapter.
3. Where, in general, are there gaps in your understanding?
4. What do you need to do to understand this process before taking the next steps in your benchmarking study?

References

1. American Productivity & Quality Center and The Healthcare Forum. *Best Practices in Hospital Admitting, Phase II.* Houston, TX: American Productivity & Quality Center and The Healthcare Forum, 1993.

2. Customer Information Center. *Quality Function Deployment for Product Definition.* Indianapolis: AT&T, 1990.

3. Customer Information Center. *Best Current Processes: Quality Function Deployment.* Indianapolis: AT&T, 1990.

4. Spendolini, M. J. *The Benchmarking Book.* New York City: AMACOM, 1992.

5. King, B. Techniques for understanding the customer. *Quality Management in Health Care* 2(2):61–67, 1994.

6. Plsek, P. Data Collection with Health Care Application. (Materials developed for the National Demonstration Project.) Roswell, GA: Paul E. Plsek & Associates, 1990.

7. Camp, R. C. *Benchmarking: The Search for Industry Best Practices That Lead to Superior Performance.* Milwaukee, WI: ASQC & Quality Resources, 1989, pp. 195 ff.

8. Kume, H. *Statistical Methods for Quality Improvement.* Adachi-ku, Japan: The Association for Overseas Technical Scholarship, 1985.

9. *Continual Improvement Handbook: A Quick Reference Guide for Tools and Concepts, Healthcare Version.* Brentwood, TN: Executive Learning, 1993.

10. American Productivity & Quality Center. *Benchmarking the Best.* Houston, TX: International Benchmarking Clearinghouse, 1993.

Phase 4: Conduct External Study

Introduction

To arrive at this point, several actions have occurred. A sponsoring organization has selected a project of enough inherent value and benefit to convince others to join in forming a benchmarking collaborative to conduct the study. These organizations have conducted the study internally, that is, among members of the collaborative. In doing so, each participant has promoted its learning, first by having developed a thorough understanding of its own process and next by having gained detailed knowledge of customer requirements. From both areas of learning participants have identified key output characteristics and key process variables. Furthermore, participants may have identified internal best practices (that is, from within the collaborative).

These practices, however, may or may not allow participants to achieve their desired level of performance. If the collaborative found and implemented best practices that further performance that meets customer requirements, members may end the project. If gaps in performance persist, the collaborative must seek opportunities outside the benchmarking collaborative for learning how to eliminate these gaps.

This chapter describes a suggested approach the collaborative and its guidance team (if it has one) can take to conduct the benchmarking project with external partners, those outside the collaborative. The following topics are included:

- How to plan for learning from external benchmarking partners
- How to conduct learning sessions with external partners
- Protocols and ethics for conducting this phase of the collaborative benchmarking model
- How to compile and analyze data gathered from outside partners
- How to develop operational improvement plans to ensure that organizations within the collaborative implement best practices learned from outside partners
- How to act on those plans to ensure that member organizations adapt the best practices and make them their own

The benchmarking strategies presented in this chapter are modeled on the Plan-Do-Study-Act (PDSA) cycle. Again, Shewhart's cycle is adopted for two reasons—its familiarity among most health care professionals involved with quality improvement and its demonstrated applicability as a model for learning and for adapting the knowledge learned. Figure 7-1 presents a graphic overview of the steps involved in the external study.

Plan

As emphasized in chapter 6, benchmarking success requires effective project planning to ensure a focus on actions that increase the likelihood of attaining

Figure 7-1. Conduct the Project with Partners Outside the Benchmarking Collaborative

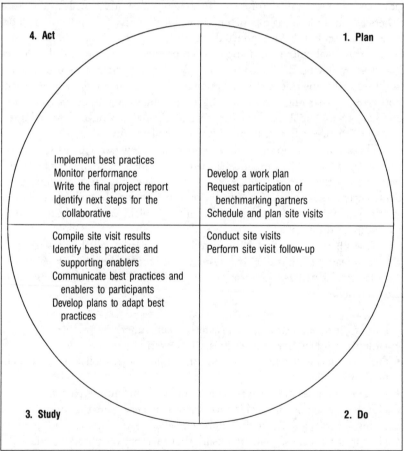

4. Act

Implement best practices
Monitor performance
Write the final project report
Identify next steps for the
    collaborative

1. Plan

Develop a work plan
Request participation of
    benchmarking partners
Schedule and plan site visits

3. Study

Compile site visit results
Identify best practices and
    supporting enablers
Communicate best practices and
    enablers to participants
Develop plans to adapt best
    practices

2. Do

Conduct site visits
Perform site visit follow-up

answers to the collaborative's questions. In addition, planning promotes efficient resource utilization to discern these key questions and to attain reliable and accurate responses to them. This section addresses specific activities associated with the Plan phase of the PDSA cycle for an external benchmarking study.

Develop a Work Plan

For the guidance team, the rationale for developing a work plan for the external portion of the study follows the same logic as that for the internal study. The plan identifies all activities to be completed, along with due dates and responsible parties. In addition, the plan helps the guidance team set forth its resource needs; provides a vehicle for communication among project stakeholders; and, most important, offers a means of measuring progress on the project.

Figure 7-2 provides a sample work plan that incorporates the steps delineated in this chapter. Some key activities that might be included in the work plan are described more fully below.

Determine What Questions to Ask

In determining what questions to ask, the collaborative can apply a variation of the essential question Joel Barker asks in his book *Future Edge*: "What is impossible to do in your business, but if it could be done, would fundamentally change it?"[1] The guidance team must ask itself "What answers, if they could be found, would propel the process to breakthrough levels of performance?"

Using this overarching question as a starting point, the guidance team brainstorms possible questions to be resolved through benchmarking with outside partners. Items on the list come from issues raised from the four areas—gaps in performance, thorough process knowledge, detailed knowledge of customer requirements, and understanding process variables and output characteristics. Once the guidance team compiles the list, it prioritizes the items to limit investigation to the few critically important questions.

An example helps show the power of knowing the right questions to ask. The joint study conducted by the Quality Improvement Networks (QINs) of The Healthcare Forum (THF) and the International Benchmarking Clearinghouse (IBC) of the American Productivity and Quality Center (APQC) examined the performance of the elective acute care inpatient admitting process. Compiling, comparing, and analyzing internal performance data from 28 participants resulted in several questions. The gaps in performance led to questions about the ability to achieve quick verification of patient eligibility for insurance coverage. Other questions raised concerned the speed with which patients were registered. These questions emanated from more detailed understanding of customer requirements.

Figure 7-2. Work Plan for Benchmarking with External Partners

July	August	September	October	November
Plan • Determine what questions to ask • Clarify the questions • Conduct primary and secondary research to identify potential partners • Screen and select partners • Develop detailed questionnaires and interview guides • Schedule and plan site visits	**Do** • Request participation • Conduct site visits • Perform site visit follow-up	**Study** • Compile site visit results • Identify best practices and supporting enablers • Communicate best practices and supporting enablers to participants	• Develop plans to adapt	**Act** • Implement adapted best practices • Monitor performance • Write final project report • Identify next steps

Clarify Questions to Ask

Before discussing *how* to clarify questions, it is necessary to understand *why* this step is important. Planning the project with partners outside the benchmarking collaborative begins with the guidance team members clarifying their understanding of the questions to be resolved. These questions arise from four possible areas:

1. *Identified gaps in performance.* Performance gaps lead to questions about why differences occur and what actions the outside partners have taken to achieve breakthrough performance.
2. *Thorough understanding of one's own process.* Process comprehension leads the guidance team to clarify questions about the processes used by outside partners.
3. *Detailed knowledge of customer requirements.* Knowing the customer allows the team to raise questions that ferret out specifics about how the external partners met similar requirements from their own customers.
4. *Comprehension of key process variables and key output characteristics.* Understanding KPVs and KOCs allows the guidance team to refine questions about relationships between variables and output characteristics of the process performed by the external partners.

Time and energy spent clarifying questions serves several purposes. First, it focuses the guidance team's line of inquiry. Benchmarking folklore tells of a company that wanted to benchmark its performance against that of a leading company. The inquiring company posed a list of about 100 questions to be discussed during the day-long site visit. This allowed for a little over four minutes per question. Such broad-based inquiry prevents detailed learning about any aspect of a process. The purpose of learning is to gain depth, not breadth. In this instance, the inquiring company was encouraged to trim its questions to a half-dozen.[2]

A second benefit is that clarifying questions helps members of the collaborative sharpen their understanding of their own process, which may lead to insights for improvement. The most important reason for ensuring clear, succinct questions is that doing so leads the guidance team in its search for external benchmarking partners that can answer the questions. It makes no sense to add a partner that cannot answer a specific question about eliminating performance gaps.

Recall that the purpose of benchmarking is to achieve breakthrough performance in areas important to the customer. Carefully formulating these questions permits effective use of resources to discern their answers while focusing the guidance team's energies. It also helps avoid "industrial tourism," the practice of conducting site visits that result in good feelings but little practical information that results in improved organizational performance.

Conduct Research to Identify Potential External Partners

Learning on the part of the collaborative depends in large part on the partners from whom it chooses to learn. Selecting the right external partners is considered by many planners to be the most difficult step in the benchmarking effort. Research sources for identifying potential external partners fall into two categories: primary and secondary. This section explores sources available to benchmarking planners so that they can make informed partner selections.

Primary Sources

Members of the collaborative and the collaborative's customers comprise primary sources. Identification of potential outside partners can begin with information from members of the collaborative (or the guidance team). An advantage of this approach is that team members have firsthand knowledge of possible candidates and their performance, as well as names of contacts within the companies who can facilitate access. There are drawbacks as well. Much of this type of information is anecdotal and subject to verification from other sources. In addition, selecting partners based on this limited information may result in partners that are personal favorites of group members but with less to offer.

Customers of the participating organizations can provide a wealth of information about other companies whose service delivery they admire. To access this source, the guidance team may need to engage in original research, such as telephone surveys specifically designed to identify those companies customers most admire. Survey results may in turn lead to focus groups to elicit responses from customers about the details of service aspects they admire. Ultimately this research effort could lead to identifying one or more of these companies as potential external partners. Again, anecdotal information should be corroborated by data drawn from secondary sources.

Secondary Sources

A detailed description of the discipline of analyzing organizations and conducting ethical competitive intelligence is beyond the scope of this text but may be found elsewhere.[3] However, using rudimentary library skills, inquiring minds, and the sources that follow, the guidance team should be able to generate a "starter" list.

- *General business press:* Much high-level information about companies and their performance can be found in business news weeklies such as *Fortune, Forbes,* and *Business Week,* which also produce periodic listings of top companies (for example "The Fortune 500," "The Forbes 400," and "The 100 Best Companies to Work for in America"). Sometimes, articles may include process-specific and performance-specific information. Due to the growing interest in benchmarking, articles may identify top performers in specific areas of performance.[4,5] (See figure 7-3.) Business textbooks may disclose innovative business practices as well as the organizations that have incorporated them into their operations.

- *Computer databases:* Computer searches may be conducted through public or university libraries or through subscription services. (See figure 7-4 for examples both within and outside of health care.)
- *Professional and trade associations, publications, and seminars:* These sources identify possible partners through articles, announcements, and workshops. They provide a way to scan for information about specific areas of performance. Because professionals in a given discipline tend to form affinity groups, the growing number of associations and societies has led to an increase in the

Figure 7-3. Some World Class Performers Identified in the Business Press

Automated inventory control
Westinghouse
Apple Computer
Federal Express

Benchmarking
Xerox
Motorola
Ford
Florida Power & Light
IBM/Rochester
DEC

Billing
American Express
MCI

Customer focus
Xerox
GE
Wallace Company
Westinghouse

Customer service
Xerox
Nordstrom, Inc.
L.L. Bean

Employee suggestions
Milliken
Dow Chemical
Toyota

Empowerment
Milliken
Honda of America

Environmental management
3M
Ben & Jerry's
Dow Chemical

Leadership
GE
Hanover Insurance
Mano, Inc.

Marketing
Helene Curtis
The Limited
Procter & Gamble
Microsoft

Product development
Motorola
DEC
Sony
3M

Purchasing
Honda
Xerox
NCR

Quality process
Westinghouse
Xerox
Toyota
IBM/Rochester

Quick changeovers
United Electric Controls
Dana Corporation
Johnson Controls

Self-directed teams
Corning
Physio Control
Toledo Scale

Training
Wallace Company
Square D

Figure 7-4. Computer Database Sources

Where to Look

- Public and university libraries
- United States Department of Commerce current industrial reports
- Washington Service Reports:
  —General Accounting Office studies
  —Congressional reports

Industrial Resources

- Key word literature searches to uncover literature resources
- Computerized databases
  —The Benchmarking Exchange
  —Dialog
  —Dun and Bradstreet
  —Standard and Poor's
  —Value Line
  —Moody's Investment Service

Health Care-Specific Resources

- Subscription services
  —HCIA
  —MedisGroups
  —CEPHIS
  —HEDIS
  —MECON PEERx Reports

---

number of articles published and number of presentations made. (See figure 7-5 for examples both within and outside of health care.)

- *Consultants, vendors, and process experts:* These sources, although less structured than others described here, provide rich insights into performance of candidate organizations. Consequently, they may require more direct contact. Ethics in benchmarking will be detailed later in the chapter, but it warrants mention here because this aspect of searching for potential partners carries with it some risk for blurring the lines of ethical business practice. Asking consultants, vendors, and process experts about the performance of other organizations may lead to misunderstanding if done inappropriately. One alternative may be to use an outside consultant to conduct this aspect of the search, thereby circumventing this concern. (See figure 7-6, p. 134.) The ethical approach to benchmarking was addressed in chapter 5.
- *Agency reports:* Reports from governmental, regulatory, and accrediting agencies may provide a cast of potential partners. For example, Form 10-K reports often contain sufficient information (auditor's statement, financial reports, bond rating, for example) from which to determine an organization's potential. Patent filings represent another potential source, as do Medicare cost reports.

Figure 7-5. Professional and Trade Associations, Publications, Seminars

Professional and Trade Associations

- American Management Association
- American Marketing Association
- American Hospital Association
- Association for Manufacturing Excellence
- The Strategic Planning Institute
- *Encyclopedia of Associations*
- American Association of Homes for the Aged

Industrial Resources

- Industry/professional journals, reports, awards
- Industry expert recommendations and forecasts
- Industry/professional association membership directories
- Speakers for industry/professional seminars and workshops
- Trade show exhibitors
- New product announcements
- Company networks

Health Care-Specific Resources

- AHA personal membership groups and directories (national and local)
- Discipline-specific membership directories (national and local)
- Awards (for example, THF Innovators Award and Young Health Care Executives)
- Speakers at national forums (for example, the Institute for Healthcare Improvement)
- Exhibitors at the American College of Healthcare Executives (ACHE) national health care congress
- Quality Management Network of the Institute for Healthcare Improvement (IHI); Quality Improvement Networks of The Healthcare Forum

In identifying outside partners, guidance teams must keep two thoughts in mind. First, the selection of partners depends on the topic being studied. Simply because a company is renowned for a particular product, outcome, or process, it does not follow that the company is a superior performer in all business dimensions. Therefore, the focus must remain on the study topic and not solely on the potential partner's reputation. Second, most benchmarking organizations can learn from *any* company that outperforms it. The approach used in the workers' compensation study is described in the following subsection.

Research Strategies: An Example

To begin the search for best-practice performers, the collaborative conducted secondary research within and outside health care. In addition to traditional library search of relevant literature, other sources included the following:

- The Risk and Insurance Management Association (RIMA)
- The Public Risk and Insurance Management Association (PRIMA)

- National Safety Council
- Occupational Safety and Health Administration (OSHA)
- Catholic Health Care Consortium (CHCC)
- Self-Insurance Institute of America
- National Commission on Compensation Insurance (NCCI)
- MMI companies

Certain sources required a more direct, personal search. The networks to which collaborative participants belong were queried to ascertain both interest and high-level performance measures. Local chapter affiliations likewise were approached. Seminar announcements were screened to identify companies and individuals who might provide leads.

This type of information led the workers' compensation benchmarking collaborative to consider outside partners in three groups—other health care systems, independent health care organizations, and premier industry performers.

Compile and Analyze Initial Information

Thus far, by analyzing key output characteristics and key process variables from member operations, the guidance team has identified crucial questions it needs

Figure 7-6. Consultants, Vendors, and Process Experts

Directories and Other Resources

- *Who's Who in Consulting*
- *Directory of Management Consultants*
- *Bradford's Directory of Market Research and Management Consultants*
- *Guide to Health Care Consultants*
- Professional associations
- Trade publication listings
- Previous organizational experience
- Referral by professional colleagues

Industrial Resources

- Industry surveys, reports
- References to individuals (press releases/announcements)
- Industry/professional association membership directories
- Speakers for industry/professional seminars and workshops
- Trade show exhibitors
- New product announcements

Health Care-Specific Resources

- *Guide to Health Care Consultants*
- Current vendors (national and local)
- Personal references from colleagues
- Speakers at national forums (for example, the Institute for Healthcare Improvement)

answered. Primary and secondary research has been conducted to identify possible benchmarking partners. Now the team must pare down the candidate list. One way to accomplish this is by gathering the known information into a data matrix, which not only allows for easy display of preliminary candidate information but also for convenience in identifying data elements missing from some companies. Also, the matrix highlights areas of differing performance.

To construct a data matrix to display comparative company performance, the guidance team begins with the KOCs and KPVs identified through its process analysis. These represent the measures against which potential external partners will be compared. Each measure is listed down the left-hand column of the matrix, and each potential partner is arrayed in its own column from left to right across the matrix. The guidance team then fills in the information for each measure under the respective company column. Once this is done the completed data matrix can assist the team in selecting those companies that perform best in the areas of interest, which in turn steers the selection of outside benchmarking partners. Figure 7-7 shows the preliminary data matrix developed for the workers' compensation study.

Novice benchmarkers may stumble at identification if they lack the secondary research skills required to conduct the search for partners. Their search may be too narrow to identify candidates with practices that provide for true breakthroughs. Failure to think in broad rather than narrow terms about the process being studied also compromises this step, a topic addressed later in this section.

An earlier discussion of prerequisites for successful benchmarking made two points that warrant reiteration here. The first relates to overcoming historical biases. If they are to succeed at benchmarking, organizations must overcome their inherent bias against learning from others. Artificial barriers built on each organization's uniqueness erode the underlying premise of benchmarking, that of collaborative learning. Benchmarking visionaries focus instead on the similarities between companies. They do so by narrowing their attention to the process that produces the results, rather than to the overall organization. By seeking commonalities, benchmarking partners find rich fields for sharing and learning. This is true even among those producing widely diverse products and services.

This willingness to learn raises the second point to be reiterated here. At this point in the collaborative benchmarking model, participants have worked with other *health care* organizations. Although minor differences may exist, most health care providers use similar processes to achieve similar results. Benchmarking with external partners raises the issue of willingness on the part of the collaborative to learn from a company that may not be in the health care field—especially if the project calls for benchmarking functions that exist outside the realm of health care (recall Ford's automobile assembly line idea from chapter 2). Therefore, the collaborative must decide whether to conduct the external study as an industry or a functional benchmarking project.

Figure 7-7. Benchmarking Partner Comparative Performance Data Matrix

Measure (KOC, KPV)*	Company Name			
	A	B	C	D
1. Experience modification factor	0.93	1.13	N/A	0.72
2. Administrative cost—percentage of total program cost	N/A	4%	N/A	3%
3. Program cost per employee	$651	$423	$700	$300
4. Incidence rate	1/8	1/9	1/12	1/6
5. Number of lost days cases per employee	0.06	0.07	0.09	0.10
6. Average lost days per lost time case	55	61	35	43
7. Cost per lost time case	$7,521	$6,702	N/A	$8,000
8. Number of claims per year	2,507	8,300	1,000	N/A
9. Percentage of medical only cases	N/A	31%	22%	16%
10. Percentage of employees on alternative duty	N/A	N/A	2%	0.1%
11.				
12.				
13.				
14.				
15.				

*Key output characteristics, key process variables

In describing types of benchmarking efforts in chapter 2, industry benchmarking was defined as identifying the best performer within a particular marketplace or within health care. This type of benchmarking focuses on the organization that performs best within a specific industry. Functional benchmarking looks across all industries to identify the company that performs best, regardless of its line of business. The topic under study plays a key role in determining which type of benchmarking effort the collaborative will conduct at this point.

For example, if the collaborative is conducting a study into best practices for performing the medical processes associated with coronary artery bypass grafts, the effort will likely be an industry benchmarking study, because no other industry performs these processes. In this case, the collaborative is restricted to learning from other health care providers and must look within the field for potential outside partners.

On the other hand, the vistas for potential outside partners broaden if the collaborative is studying an administrative, financial, support, or human resources function. Many companies perform the same processes to achieve fundamentally the same result. In the financial area, for example, most companies perform billing and accounts receivable processes. Every company with employees uses a process to recruit and hire personnel. All companies have a distribution system to move products within the company and out to customers. Because of these similarities, opportunities to conduct functional benchmarking studies with outside partners expand as the collaborative considers topics beyond direct, hands-on patient care.

The lesson here is for the collaborative to think broadly, or generically, about the process so as to expand opportunities for finding external partners. The adaptation of industrial laser technology for medical purposes exemplifies the application of broader thinking. Observing a technology clearly superior to present methods, recognizing its generic nature, and modifying it to one's own setting is at the heart of this learning. Several factors determine whether the collaborative conducts industry or functional benchmarking.

Topic

The project topic is the key determinant of the type of study undertaken. If the topic lends itself to study across industries, a functional benchmarking effort may be warranted but only if the project is a general business function or can be viewed in generic terms. Practitioners observe that "practices found in dissimilar industries are more readily accepted [by management and workers] than those within the same industry."[6] Therefore the opportunities for breakthrough may be greater.

Likelihood of Participation

Businesses outside health care may not see the relevance of particular patient care topics. Yet, they may willingly participate in studies more germane to their own operations. Because most companies rely on support and administrative processes (such as logistics, transportation, staff acquisitions, and bill paying), non-health care businesses may be more willing to participate in benchmarking projects.

Cost

The relative costs of conducting an industry versus a functional study is a key consideration. Study costs depend as much on the number and location of partners selected as on the type of study.

Consider Four Crucial Elements

Before the guidance team can identify appropriate partners, at least four elements must be taken into account. These are the degree of improvement needed.

the number of partners needed, the characteristic to be investigated, and the time required to search for potential partners.

How Much Improvement?

The degree of improvement needed influences the search for possible partners. If the collaborative requires improvement in orders of magnitude, it may need to undertake a broad search for partners to find adequate best practices to achieve the level of performance desired. The desire to find the best of the best must be balanced against the likelihood of gaining that company's participation and the cost of conducting that portion of the study; no formula can assess this balance, only the collective judgment of guidance team members. Remember, the larger the net used to scroll for partners, the greater the likelihood of identifying possible performance breakthroughs.

How Many Partners?

More than one partner may be needed. Mature benchmarkers recognize that no one company is superior at every aspect of a process. For example, in benchmarking the elective acute care inpatient admitting process, one partner was proficient at speedy registration but had no experience with insurance verification procedures and consequently sought another partner for insights into that portion of the process. The "right" number of partners is that number necessary to answer the questions raised by the guidance team.

What to Investigate?

By knowing the fundamental characteristic (process feature) it wishes to improve, the collaborative expands its list of candidates for partnership. In their books, Camp and Balm respectively provide excellent examples of how benchmarking teams thought beyond the narrow scope of routine thinking to identify the fundamental characteristics the teams sought to improve.[7,8] Figure 7-8 is a brief summary adapted from their examples.

Figure 7-8. Examples of Thinking Generically about Processes

If a fundamental characteristic is:	A potential industry partner will be:
Inventory turnover	Perishable goods (e.g., produce, flowers)
Fast customer service	Fast-food chain, selected retail services
Ultrahigh reliability	Aerospace firm, surgical implants specialist
Minimizing high risk	Farming, high-risk insurance carrier, movie stunts

Adapted from R. C. Camp, *Benchmarking: The Search for Industry Best Practices That Lead to Superior Performance,* and G. J. Balm, *Benchmarking: A Practitioner's Guide for Becoming and Staying Best of the Best.*

Applying this thinking to health care, assume a medical center is working to decrease the time required to obtain laboratory results for emergency room patients. Specifically this example is about laboratory test result response time; more generally, it is about turnaround time. Thinking in generic terms allows for a wider range of potential comparisons and learning from more diverse companies. Many of these companies perform processes generically the same as those the benchmarking collaborative is studying.

How Much Time to Conduct the Search?
Identifying potential outside benchmarking partners requires a time investment for research into sources beyond those immediately available to the collaborative. This research often requires exploration of multiple sources so that the guidance team can home in on viable candidates. A potential disadvantage with multiple sources is conflicting information; for example, one outside source might report on a company's activities favorably whereas another might look on that same performance with disfavor or indifference. It is incumbent on the benchmarking collaborative to allow sufficient time to resolve such conflicts (as discussed later in this chapter). Time requirements will vary with the project topic, available resources, range of partner candidates, and whether the study is an industry or functional benchmarking project.

Screen and Select Outside Partners

The guidance team (or benchmarking collaborative) is now ready to screen potential partners and make its selection. Screening follows from the information gathered through primary and secondary research. The guidance team uses the data matrix to provide objective analysis of potential partners. To select the right partners, the team must consider several critical factors and examine key questions about those companies.

Screening Potential Partners
The screening of potential partners is driven by the nature of the project and by the nature of each participant in the collaborative. To screen effectively, the team should explore responses to the following questions:

1. Have the processes been operable in the company long enough to demonstrate a proven track record?
2. Have substantial and successful process improvements that are quantifiable or measurable been made?
3. Do the potential partners represent sufficiently different industries or organizations to increase the likelihood for identifying best practices and providing ample opportunity for learning?

4. Do the companies represented demonstrate innovative and successful processes?
5. Do the companies demonstrate ethical behavior consistent with the specifications of the collaborative?

The research conducted by the group should provide the answers to these
questions. If that is not the case, the guidance team may seek additional sources.

Watson suggests four questions the guidance team may wish to add when
considering which companies to use as partners.[9] These questions have been
paraphrased here to reflect their applicability in a benchmarking collaborative:

1. Does the guidance team have sufficient information to indicate that a superior
   performance difference exists?
2. How recent and reliable is the information about this company?
3. Would any differences in the business of this potential partner invalidate
   the comparison or pose a barrier to the information?
4. Is this company likely to share the details of its process with the collaborative?

Cost, time, and access may be added as implicit considerations. For example,
a company might meet all four criteria, but the cost and time to gain access
to it may eliminate that company as a viable candidate.

Such considerations hold implications for the guidance team during this
assessment. The group must be sensitive to the differing perspectives of its
members—a company might meet the criteria for partnership but compete
directly with a member of the collaborative, for example. Such a scenario might
mean dropping the company from consideration. The collaborative will be better
served if such sensitivities are identified in advance and dealt with appropriately. Such actions also will save time and resources by reducing falsely identified partners.

Selecting Partners

When does the guidance team know when it has selected the right partners?
No algorithm measures the accuracy of this decision at this point in the project.
Only at project completion, when the collaborative has learned and adapted
best practices, can it make this determination. Until that time, the group must
rely on the preliminary data gathered, analysis of those data, and its collective
judgment about potential partners.

The guidance team may wish to limit the number of partners to six to
eight. This provides a varied but manageable number while reducing the difficulties incurred with massive data gathering and analysis. However, the team must
keep in mind that the number of partners must be sufficient to answer the
questions raised by the process analysis.

Each outside partner may be able to answer several questions whereas some
may be capable of responding only in one area. The potential for multiple views

on issues important to the collaborative increases the likelihood for identifying an adaptable best practice for collaborative members.

Develop Questionnaires and Interview Guides

Once the guidance team has identified outside partners, it must develop specific questionnaires and interview guides to steer benchmarking sessions. The purpose of these sessions is to gather as much useful information as possible about details of the partner's process. The guidance team should do this with minimal disruption and inconvenience to the partner.

Three vehicles can accomplish this information gathering: written surveys, telephone interviews, and site visits. Surveys may be mailed, sent via facsimile copier, or transmitted directly from one computer terminal to another.

Written Surveys

Written surveys are appropriate if the information to be gathered is general and statistical in nature, rather than process focused. Surveys allow more data to be gathered from more partners, but such data often lack consistency and/or supporting background information. On the other hand, survey data may lend themselves to comparative data analysis if the level of information is sufficient to determine how best practices operate. Studies that utilize only written surveys run the risk of becoming comparative data analyses only and not true benchmarking studies. In the context of benchmarking studies, written surveys most often provide a further understanding of partners. For example, additional contact, either through telephone interviews or site visits, may be needed to clarify knowledge of the process and practices behind what the data reveal.

Telephone Interviews

Telephone interviews present an alternative to surveys that bring the advantage of interactive dialogue. They also increase the level of participation among targeted audiences because they are typically shorter and more focused than written surveys. Telephone interviews allow the guidance team to query the specifics of a process in the partner's operation with those intimately involved with it. Phone calls also permit participants to seek support information immediately whenever questions need to be clarified. Telephone interviews, however, cannot overcome the drawback of absence of direct observation of the process in operation, a requirement in some benchmarking projects.

Questionnaire Development

Regardless of whether written surveys, telephone interviews, or site visits are used, the guidance team must develop questions that will yield the information sought from interviews. The answers to these questions will lead the team to uncover the partner's best practices which, when adapted into operation, will lead to breakthrough process performance sought by the collaborative. To maximize its learning from partners, the guidance team needs to focus its inquiry through effective questionnaire design.[10]

Toward this end, the team is concerned with two issues—*relevance* and *accuracy* of information. Obtaining only that information germane to the study topic will keep the discussion concentrated. Doing so serves both the collaborative and the partner: The guidance team is served by gaining a wealth of pertinent information about how to solve its performance problems, and the partner is served by having its time respected by the guidance team. Sessions with partners are not fishing expeditions; they are structured opportunities for learning specific practices.

Ensuring accuracy entails verifying information as it is gathered. It may require asking the same question different ways to gain perspectives on responses.

The guidance team needs to structure inquiries for outside benchmarking partners as *open-ended questions*, which are designed to encourage dialogue between the parties. Such questions promote discussion of topics that are important to both and relevant to the process under study.

Questions should be phrased clearly, avoiding industry-specific terminology, jargon, and abbreviations. They should be few in number (up to 10) and focus on the key aspects of the process that the benchmarking partner can explain to the guidance team.

In asking questions, the guidance team must be sensitive to its host benchmarking partner. No question should embarrass the partner. Likewise, no information should be sought that the collaborative would not want to share of its own. Figure 7-9 lists sample questions to be asked of a benchmarking partner in the workers' compensation benchmarking study.

Request Participation of Benchmarking Partners

Having identified and selected external partners, the collaborative is ready to enter the next arena of learning, to request formal participation from the partners. This

Figure 7-9. Sample Questions to Ask a Benchmarking Partner

1. Given your strong performance of this process, what have you identified as key variables contributing to your performance?

2. What supports or other considerations have been helpful to you in attaining such consistently high performance in this area?

3. What barriers did you overcome to achieve this high level of performance? How did you overcome them?

4. What lessons have you learned about this process that you applied to other processes?

5. What recommendations do you have if we were to try to adapt your practices into our own process?

is accomplished using a simple letter of request for participation sent by the guidance team to the chosen partners. The letter, which should be addressed to the quality executive or the line manager of the process, should explain the benchmarking collaborative, its composition, and its purpose. The request should focus on the narrow points of interest within the particular partner. For example, when a collaborative is working with an external benchmarking partner to examine how claims are managed in workers' compensation, their request should focus on specific activities taken by that partner to perform the claims management process exceptionally well. They may focus on document handling as a specific activity. If possible, the request should include a preliminary set of the questions the guidance team wants answered by each partner.

The letter should advise the recipient that someone from the guidance team will follow up with a telephone call (within a stated time frame) to answer any questions the partner may have. This follow-up phone call is also an opportunity for the guidance team to determine if the letter reached the appropriate individual and if there is a sufficient level of interest in participating in the project.

Following the initial letter with a call fulfills two key principles of organizational communications.[11] One, message redundancy reinforces message retention. Two, the use of several media is more effective than the use of just one. The second principle can be taken a step further with an office visit, if logistics permit.

The importance of sending the letter to the right person cannot be stressed enough. The worst that can happen if the letter goes to the wrong person is that the request may be immediately dismissed as irrelevant. At best, action on the request may be delayed while the right party is sought. Neither should happen if secondary research has been done adequately.

The guidance team should already have recognized that it will operate on the partners' timetable, not its own. To the extent that the collaborative depends on the partners for learning, it must temper its own schedule to accommodate that of partners. As a result, this stage of the project may not proceed as the collaborative might like—but such is the nature of learning ventures. Figure 7-10 provides a sample letter of request for participation in the workers' compensation benchmarking study.

Schedule and Plan Site Visits

Site visits provide a way around lack of direct observation of a process, mainly through direct contact with partners. Visits allow observers to see not only the process but the environment in which the process operates. The disadvantage of site visits is their costs, which depend on distance and the number of team members participating in the visit. Site visits cost more than other forms of interactions with partners, but typically they generate the most benefit as well. If the process being studied requires direct observation to learn the best practices, few options prove more beneficial than site visits.

As with all other aspects of the work plan, preparation contributes to a successful site visit by creating the proper environment and attitude. Before significant sharing can occur, rapport between the parties must be established. Building rapport begins with the initial contact and continues through the site visit and follow-up conversations. Long-term relationships built through benchmarking can perpetuate breakthroughs for all parties involved.

Figure 7-10. Sample Letter Requesting Participation by a Benchmarking Partner

Date

Company Contact
Title
Company
Street
City, State Zipcode

Company contact:

Our organization is undertaking a study of the best workers' compensation practices companies use today. We were directed to you through our research into companies that perform workers' compensation claims management particularly well. Several sources cited your company as one that manages claims consistently better than most.

Within our corporation, a benchmarking collaborative has been formed to identify and adapt the best practices in workers' compensation. Ten health care providers compose that benchmarking collaborative, including hospitals and long-term care organizations. They have come together to collectively learn the best ways to improve their performance in workers' compensation claims management.

Because your organization is consistently cited as one of the best performers, we'd like the opportunity to learn from your experience. We'd like to schedule a site visit within the next two months between representatives from our benchmarking collaborative and from your staff. The purpose of that meeting is to discuss specific details of your claims process that allow it to perform so admirably. A brochure describing our organization and some material on the collaborative accompany this letter. In addition, I've included a listing of the topics the team would like to discuss with you while on-site.

Our team will include four people. Three of these individuals represent some aspect of the claims process. The fourth is our internal benchmarking team facilitator.

I will call you in about two weeks to determine what additional information I can provide to allow you to positively consider this request. At that time, I'll try to answer any questions you might have.

Thank you in advance for considering our request.

Sincerely,

Workers' Compensation Benchmarking Team Leader

Assuming the guidance team will contact several outside benchmarking partners, it needs a mechanism to ensure that these sessions create the right impression and run smoothly. A scheduling matrix helps coordinate activities to ensure flawless contacts. A sample scheduling matrix is presented in figure 7-11. This format, adapted from the work of AT&T, presents an easy way for the guidance team to track its preparation for site visits.[12]

Before site visits are confirmed, members of the guidance team should assign responsibilities for activities to ensure their completion. Those activities include negotiations about logistics of the visit; correspondence (requesting, confirming, and follow-up letters); information packet; notes during the visit; and report of the visit. In addition, role assignments during the site visit should be confirmed among team members. Typically, three roles emerge—interviewer, observer, and documenter. The interviewer asks questions of the partner and steers the discussion; the observer watches for behavior tips (for example, body language) beyond what is actually answered; and the documenter takes notes and later compiles the information shared during the visit. These assignments can be incorporated into the scheduling matrix.

The team needs to be sure that it obtains the necessary approvals well in advance of the site visits. This approval should come from both the collaborative and outside partners. Again, scheduling site visits is at the convenience of partners. Once approvals have been received and logistics determined, letters confirming arrangements should be sent. Confirming letters also should include information packets about the collaborative and its purpose. If preliminary questions were not sent with the letter requesting participation, they should be sent with the confirming letter. The guidance team should be sure that all its members receive the same information that is sent to the outside partners.

Shortly before the scheduled site visit, each partner should be telephoned to confirm arrangements again. This anticipates any last-minute changes in individual participants or logistics. It also reassures all parties that the stage is set for the upcoming visit.

Those attending the site visits should be selected based on their knowledge of the particular process aspect under study, as well as their ability to perform one of the three roles described. For example, if the site visit team is to learn best practices in insurance verification as part of the admitting process, those with the most intimate knowledge of this area should participate. Keeping the size of the site visit team to a manageable number prevents overwhelming the benchmarking partner with an entourage, and it helps keep site visit costs under control.

Do

Having completed the planning and preparation activities, the guidance team is ready to conduct site visits to the outside benchmarking partners it selected.

Figure 7-11. Benchmarking Partner Scheduling Matrix

	Companies			
	A	**B**	**C**	**D**
Benchmarking partner				
Address				
Contact person				
Telephone				

Site visit attendees:
  Partner
  Collaborative				

Site visit:
  Date
  Time
  Locale				

Travel logistics				

Preparation responsibilities:
  Correspondence
  Confirmation
  Logistics
  Information packet				

On-site responsibilities:
  Interviewer
  Observer
  Documenter				

Comments				
Other				

Adapted from: *Benchmarking: Focus on World-Class Practices.* Indianapolis: AT&T Bell Laboratories Technical Publications Center, 1992, p. 111.

To accomplish this Do phase of the project effectively, the team must perform two groups of activities: conduct site visits in a manner consistent with ethical guidelines and protocols, and perform follow-up activities to ensure effective use of information gathered and continued goodwill of external partners.

Conduct Site Visits

The site visit provides opportunities for the guidance team to learn firsthand from their chosen partners. Out of respect for the benchmarking partner's time, these sessions should start and end on time. The agenda for the session should be developed in advance jointly by the guidance team and the partner. Following an agenda ensures that both parties have allocated time adequately to learn the information sought. As in all project efforts to date, the visit is facilitated by honest, professional, and courteous behaviors.

The visit should begin with introductions and a brief explanation of why each person is at the session and the perspective he or she brings. Before addressing specifics of the visit, locations of rest rooms, telephones, coat rooms, and the like should be announced.

Observe the organizational culture of the hosting organization. For example, use first or last names and titles, as the host does. Follow the seating patterns of the host. Pay particular attention to the serving of beverages and meals, as these reveal much about an organization's culture. These artifacts of organizational culture demonstrate its values and may display some cultural enablers that encourage superior process performance.

Provide a brief overview of the project, clarifying the objectives of the overall effort and describing the approach used to bring the collaborative to this point. Explain why this organization was selected as a benchmarking partner, including the information that led to selection.

Begin with general, open-ended questions and work toward more specific ones. Maintain focus on questions and information pertinent to the objectives and the process being studied. Address one question at a time. If a question is not answered to the satisfaction of the team, seek clarification by rephrasing the question. To minimize any confusion caused by language differences across industries, use general or universal terminology, avoiding industry jargon and abbreviations. For example, representatives may not understand "UB-82," but they will understand universal billing form.

Stick to the team roles identified prior to the visit—interviewer, observer, and documenter. Orchestrate the guidance team's questions so only one person speaks at a time. Share information from the process studied by the benchmarking collaborative. If appropriate, offer to share the results of the entire effort, pending agreement by all partners involved. Offer to facilitate a reciprocal visit, if the partner appears interested. Create the opportunity for follow-up questions and additional benchmarking projects in the future.

Finish the session on time. Thank the partner for the time, information, and insights. Figure 7-12 is a site visit checklist of key activities.

Figure 7-12. Site Visit Checklist

_____ Develop agenda jointly with benchmarking partner

_____ Follow agenda

_____ Introduce participants:
  From collaborative
  From benchmarking partner

_____ Explain each person's reason for attending

_____ Identify locations of rest rooms, telephones, closets

_____ Follow the lead of the hosting organization's use of titles, names, and seating arrangements

_____ Explain the project purpose and objectives

_____ Describe the approach used to bring the collaborative to this point in the study

_____ Identify why this particular benchmarking partner was selected

_____ Begin with general, open-ended questions; follow up with more specific ones

_____ Address one question at a time; seek clarification as necessary

_____ Use general, universal language

_____ Adhere to the roles identified: interviewer, observer, documenter

_____ Offer to share results of the entire effort, subject to the approval of all parties

_____ Offer to host a reciprocal site visit for the partner

Perform Site Visit Follow-Up

Upon returning from each site visit, the conducting team has several tasks to accomplish. First, it must send a thank-you letter to the benchmarking partner, reiterating its thanks and keeping the door open for additional questions and follow-up. (See figure 7-13.)

The team should schedule a time to debrief as soon as possible after the site visit. This allows the team to identify essential elements of its learning about performance measures, process attributes, and the environment of the benchmarking partner. If the geographic dispersion of the collaborative presents a challenge on this score, it can be met through conducting the briefing via structured conference call.

The site visit team also must write a site visit report. This report should follow a prescribed format that allows the reports from different site visits to be compiled and compared more easily. The format content may be similar to that on the scheduling matrix shown in figure 7-11 (p. 146). In addition to "boilerplate" information, the group needs to capture the questions asked and the responses given. Figure 7-14 presents a sample format for documenting a site visit report.

Figure 7-13. Sample Thank-You Letter

Date

Company Contact
Title
Company
Street
City, State Zipcode

Dear _____,

Thank you for your gracious hospitality during our recent benchmarking site visit.
I appreciate the care you took to make the visit a successful experience for our team.
Please extend our thanks to all the members of your team who contributed their time and
energies to make our learning such a pleasurable experience. Offer our special thanks to
Ms. X, who coordinated our collective efforts.

The information you shared will prove invaluable to us as we formulate changes to our
workers' compensation process. The practices you incorporate into your process should
help us improve our own efforts.

We anticipate continuing dialogue among those who attended the benchmarking site visit.
This ongoing exchange of ideas will help us move forward to implement a model process
for workers' compensation.

Again, thank you for your help and hospitality. We look forward to our future discussions.

Sincerely,

Workers' Compensation Benchmarking Team Leader

Figure 7-14. Sample Site Visit Report and Discussion Format

Benchmarking partner:	Company name hosting visit
Address:	Location
Contact person:	Key partner representative
Site visit attendees:	
Partner:	Hosting company representatives
Collaborative:	Members conducting site visit
Site visit date:	Date
Background:	Relevant information about hosting company and reasons why it was selected as partner, including both measures and practices
Key findings:	High-level, germane information gleaned from site visit; include both statistical information and observations; focus on items critical to partner's success
Q&A:	More detail of the above; structured around specific questions asked by site visit team and responses provided by the partner
Discussion points:	Highlights of discussion among collaborative members about this site visit and findings; includes any added insights generated by group

The site visit team also must discuss the results of the site visit with those members of the collaborative who did not participate in the site visit. This communication shares the team's impressions of the partner, as well as insights and knowledge gained. The group may wish to document this discussion in a standardized format, with essential points of discussion captured in outline format that lists both hard and soft data. This provides an opportunity to identify the cultural aspects of the visit, in case they impinge on process performance. The format provided in figure 7-14 also can be adapted for documenting this discussion. Here, too, the geographic dispersion of the collaborative may require use of teleconferencing or electronic mail.

Study

The Study portion of the PDSA cycle reveals lessons learned by the collaborative and site visit teams. To organize these lessons and make them more readily available for use by the collaborative, several activities must occur. First, the guidance team must compile the information obtained from the site visits into a common and easy-to-use format and then identify best practices and supporting enablers. Next, the group communicates these findings to the participating organizations so that they can develop plans to adapt these best practices into their respective operations.

Compile Site Visit Results

To follow up on site visits, the guidance team must compile meaningful statistical results, as well as supporting narrative information that explains the data in a useful format. The format should promote effective comparison and analysis of information from the different site visits.

Compilation requires the guidance team to organize the performance measures and process attributes into a data matrix. Continuing the example of the workers' compensation study, figure 7-15 presents a sample format for a benchmarking partner comparative analysis that incorporates key outcome characteristics and key process variables as base measures for the study. The format allows space for the guidance team to identify and document the best practices observed from site visits. In addition, the format permits space for listing enablers the teams identified during site visits.

Recall from an earlier discussion that enablers are elements in the organizational infrastructure that allow the best practice to occur. For example, if a best practice is the speedy admission of patients directly to their rooms, this process innovation is enabled by two information system supports. First, the admitting staff person on the nursing unit must have access to computers with which to gather the necessary financial, demographic, and clinical information. This element enables the admission to be performed on the unit, away from an

Figure 7-15. Benchmarking Partner Comparative Analysis

	Partner			
	A	**B**	**C**	**D**
Key Outcome Characteristics:				
Claims incidence rate				
Percent lost days cases				
Experience modification				
Cost per lost day case				
% Administrative cost				
Key Process Variables:				
Time to first contact				
Claims resolution				
Best Practices:				
Contact				
Follow-up				
Claims filing				
Reporting				
Case management				
Enablers:				
Information system				
Medical staff relations				
Safety & prevention				

admitting department. Second, a database of patient information enables the patient to *verify* rather than *reiterate* information previously given. Although not best practices in and of themselves, these elements are enablers—they allow best practices to occur.

Identify Best Practices and Supporting Enablers

The guidance team can identify best practices and enablers only by discussing the results of the site visits among the group. This structured discussion helps organize the findings and experiences of teams that conducted the site visits. In these sessions, participants examine external partner responses to questions, additional data gathered by team members, and impressions the team formed during site visits. Although each site visit team will likely provide anecdotes about their visits, the discussion should focus on the process under study and the practices observed, relating these practices to results achieved and identifying outcomes that stand out as superior.

Once best practices have been identified, the group can discuss the elements that reside in those companies that enable the best practices to flourish. The discussion of enablers must always be related back to the best practices. Sometimes team members are tempted to define something as an enabler simply because it represents a new technology. Remember, an enabler links directly to the best practice it supports.

Communicate Best Practices and Enablers to Participants

After identifying best practices encountered in its search and enablers that support them, the guidance team now has the responsibility to communicate these findings to the collaborative. This report briefly describes the practices, their supporting enablers, respective sources, and any supplemental information that might help participating organizations determine applicability of the best practice in their settings.

Develop Plans to Adapt Best Practices

Once the guidance team identifies the list of best practices and enablers, each organization within the collaborative must assess how those best practices fit with current organizational operations. This is accomplished through analyzing how the best practices can be melded with the existing process. Whether this requires adapting the best practices, process redesign, or developing a new process depends on how the current process is performing. Once again applying the PDSA model, the teams charged with implementing the changes within participating organizations will use a four-step approach to improvement initiatives. First teams *plan* the improvement. Next, they implement (*do*) the improvement on a pilot basis. Third, they *study* the results of the pilot to be sure those results provide the needed improvement. Finally, they *act* to institutionalize the improvement throughout the organization.

The implementation plans of each organization in the collaborative must be tailored precisely to the needs of the organization and the scope of changes needed in the process in order to meet customer requirements. Again, the scope of changes may range from adaptation of observed best practices for fit into the existing process; to redesign of the existing process, incorporating many of the demonstrated best practices; to design of a wholly new process, based on the learning of best practices.

The scope of changes depends on two factors – the gap between current performance and customer requirements, and capability of the process. If the gap is small, adapting only some of the best practices may allow the process to perform adequately. If the gap is significant, the process may require more extensive redesign or a completely new design. Similarly, the capability of the process dictates whether merely incorporating best practices or replacing the process is called for.

For example, after working with outside benchmarking partners on a project conducted on the admitting process, the organization discovers that the gap between its performance and that of the benchmark performer, as measured by average admitting time, is more than one hour. Further, the organization discovers that its own process, no matter how much improvement is measured, seems incapable of admitting patients in less than 20 minutes on average. Given this substantial gap in service and the likelihood that the current process is incapable of meeting benchmark performance through incremental improvement, a process redesign or replacement is called for.

Once the scope of process changes has been identified, the team identifies resource needs (money, time, personnel) and then assigns responsibility for implementing the changes within the designated time frame using the resources allowed. The plan should specify the systems, tools, skills, and support necessary to make the changes successfully. In addition, the team should design methods for communicating with stakeholders of the process. To ensure that changes happen in a timely way, the team should place milestones in the plan so as to monitor progress of implementation.

Act

Before beginning process changes, benchmarking teams in each organization share their plans with various stakeholders of the process. This sharing occurs through existing communication vehicles that help gain understanding and acceptance on the part of stakeholders. Regularly scheduled management and staff meetings provide opportunities to inform them of planned changes, as do written communications such as newsletters and employee mailings. Existing channels allow the team to communicate benefits of the benchmarking effort with key constituents of the organization.

Implement Best Practices

Once the organizational team has discussed its plans with the proper groups, it is prepared to begin implementation. Implementation is accomplished through the Plan-Do-Study-Act cycle that is part of the organization's quality initiative and a guide for systematic improvement. As described earlier, the team implementing the changes in the participating organization applies the PDSA cycle used in its organization's quality improvement process: *plan* the improvement, *do* the improvement on a pilot basis, *study* pilot results to be sure they achieve the degree of improvement needed, and *act* to standardize the improvement throughout the organization.

Monitor Performance

Performance monitoring allows the team implementing improvements to select measures of performance appropriate for the improved process. These measures, which reflect both outcomes and process measures, ideally monitor performance of key process variables and assess key output characteristics. For example, a team implementing improvements in the workers' compensation process may choose to monitor the number of lost days per case and experience modification factors as key output characteristics (experience modification factors are adjustments made to an organization's insurance rates, based on previous years' experience). It also may monitor claims processing time as a key process variable.

Performance monitoring assesses whether planned gains occurred. Measurements that result from this monitoring tell whether the gains have held and provide input for future continuous improvement activities.

Write the Final Project Report

Once members of the collaborative have developed their plans and launched improvement efforts, the guidance team is positioned to draft a report on the project. The purpose of this report is to communicate the approach used, lessons learned, and process changes identified. Because it will be written before the process changes have been carried out fully, the report can only recount the experiences of the collaborative. Figure 7-16 presents a possible outline for this report. In addition to documenting lessons learned—not only for this project but for the collaborative as well—the report captures lessons about working cooperatively, lessons that can be applied in other group settings and with other projects.

Identify Next Steps for the Collaborative

Once the collaborative completes its report to members, it has fulfilled its purpose of bringing together organizations seeking to improve performance in a process commonly agreed on. It identified best practices in that process from

Figure 7-16. Sample Outline for Project Report

I. Introduction
   A. Overview
   B. Report format
II. Project sponsor
   A. Organization demographics
III. Process under study
   A. Rationale for selection
   B. Boundaries on scope of project
IV. Participants in the collaborative
   A. Organization demographics
   B. Individuals involved
V. Approach/model used
   A. Overview of methodology
   B. Identification of sentinel events
VI. Compilation of current process performance
   A. Questionnaires/instruments used
   B. Summary level data
   C. Conclusions/observations
VII. Best practices found within the collaborative
   A. Rationale for selection
   B. Information sources
VIII. Recap of site visits
   A. Company specific summary
   B. Characteristics
IX. Best practices found among benchmarking partners
   A. Rationale for selection
   B. Key elements of practices
   C. Enablers
X. Implementation plans
   A. Highlights from participants' implementation plans
   B. Planned follow-up
XI. Next steps
   A. Future efforts

among the group and learned from that experience. The collaborative then turned its attention externally to learn from other companies that perform a similar process. From these learning experiences, the collaborative identified best practices and adapted them as their own. Finally, the collaborative compiled a report to the member organizations, recounting the experience and the benefits participants derived from it. The collaborative has two remaining responsibilities: assessing progress and looking to the future.

Assessing Adaptation and Implementation Progress

To complete its accountability to improve performance in the process selected for the current project, the collaborative may schedule periodic assessments to monitor performance improvements. If members agree, assessments can be conducted annually (for example) to determine how much of the planned adaptation and implementation have occurred. Periodic assessments offer two benefits. First, they stimulate continued attention to the process studied by giving participants added incentive to carry out the process changes as planned. Second, and more important, regular evaluation allows members to share additional learning about performance improvements.

Looking to the Future

The collaborative has traveled through stages common to team development and formed relationships that encourage sharing and learning. Now that the project is completed, members must either adjourn the collaborative upon acceptance of the project report or move to another project. If the group chooses to conduct another benchmarking project, the approach described in this text is repeated, beginning with project selection.

Summary

This chapter described how a benchmarking study can be conducted with partners outside the collaborative. This final phase of the collaborative model for benchmarking in health care utilizes the PDSA framework established in chapter 6, again drawing on its familiarity among quality professionals and building on their experience with quality improvement initiatives in their organizations.

The PDSA cycle also offers the advantage of being an approach based on scientific inquiry and disciplined learning. Applied in the context of a benchmarking model, the cycle permits the collaborative to work with external partners to identify best practices for adaptation into the collaborative's own organizations. Learning from others and using that knowledge to improve its health care service delivery is the bottom-line goal of forming collaborative partnerships with other facilities.

Upon completing this phase of the model, the collaborative examines its own future. It may reconvene to assess progress made by participants in implementing adapted best practices. The group may also choose either to work on another project of mutual interest, applying the same model, or simply disband.

Putting These Ideas to Work

Objective

Identify and list secondary research sources you could use to identify potential outside benchmarking partners.

Approach

1. Pose the brainstorming question: "What sources do we have for identifying potential outside benchmarking partners for the project we have
   selected?"
2. Be as specific when creating this list. Ask each participant to respond
   to the question by writing one source on a sticky note. Allow time (perhaps
   10 minutes) for participants to consider their response.
3. Gather responses in a round-robin, requesting individuals to post their
   sticky notes on the wall.
4. Eliminate duplications.
5. Sort the remaining sources into groups. Participants may define the groups
   in advance or use an affinity diagram to identify them.
6. Assign participants the task of using these sources to identify potential
   external partners.

References and Notes

1. Barker, J. A. *Future Edge: Discovering the New Paradigms of Success.* New York City:
   Morrow, 1992, p. 147.

2. Heidbreder, J. E. Benchmarking, the Success Analysis Tool. Presentation at annual
   meeting of The Healthcare Forum, Anaheim, CA, Apr. 12, 1992.

3. Fuld, L. M. *Competitor Intelligence: How to Get It, How to Use It.* New York City:
   John F. Wiley, 1985. This text provides detailed insights into the ways to identify
   secondary sources for competitive intelligence and provides directions on how to
   gather and use it in ethical ways.

4. Altany, D. Copycats. *Industry Week* 239(21):11–18, Nov. 5, 1990.

5. Altany, D. Share and share alike. *Industry Week* 240(14):12–13, July 15, 1991.

6. Camp, R. C. *Benchmarking: The Search for Industry Best Practices That Lead to Superior
   Performance.* Milwaukee: ASQC Quality Press, 1989, p. 62.

7. Camp, p. 65.

8. Balm, G. J. *Benchmarking: A Practitioner's Guide for Becoming and Staying Best of the
   Best.* Schaumburg, IL: QPMA Press, 1992, p. 85.

9. Watson, G. H. *The Benchmarking Workbook: Adapting Best Practices for Performance
   Improvement.* Cambridge, MA: Productivity Press, 1992, pp. 54–56.

10. Zikmund, W. G. *Business Research Methods.* Chicago: The Dryden Press, 1991, pp.
    297–326. This text provides a fuller discussion of considerations in questionnaire
    design.

11. Klein, S. M. Communication strategies for successful organizational change. *Indus-
    trial Management* 36(1):26, Jan./Feb., 1994.

12. AT&T Benchmarking Team. *Benchmarking: Focus on World-Class Practices.* Indianapolis:
    AT&T Bell Laboratories Technical Publications Center, 1992, p. 111.

Chapter Eight

Managing the Benchmarking Team

Introduction

Benchmarking is accomplished through teamwork—a critical variable in the effect benchmarking has on learning and performance. Teamwork is necessary in every phase of the collaborative model, from selecting the study topic, through understanding internal work processes, to implementing best practices. Teams mobilize resources for establishing the collaborative, helping members understand how processes work, documenting customer requirements, collecting data, studying best practices, and discovering creative ways to adapt those best practices into work processes in order to achieve breakthrough results. Within this context, teams are the medium through which organizations learn.

Having laid out a rationale for benchmarking in health care, provided a collaborative model for finding and implementing best practices, and delineated the steps in collaborative benchmarking, attention now turns to management of the benchmarking team. This chapter describes important characteristics of a benchmarking team, variables in team success, roles within the team, developmental stages of the benchmarking team, training requirements for team members, and why teamwork is emphasized as a process for organizational learning.

Benchmarking Team Characteristics

In practice, collaborative benchmarking involves teams at two levels: the benchmarking team in each participating organization and the team (usually the guidance team) that conducts the external study for the collaborative. Throughout this chapter, the term *team* refers to either entity.

Benchmarking teams and quality improvement (QI) teams share a common set of characteristics. Figure 8-1 depicts the dimensions that the benchmarking team generally shares with improvement teams: purpose, leadership, membership, training, procedures, dynamics, and duration.

Figure 8-1. Characteristics of Benchmarking Teams Compared with CQI Teams

	Benchmarking Team	QI Team
Purpose	Find and implement best practices to achieve breakthrough results	Improving processes
Leadership	Process owner; perhaps co-owner or alternate	Process owner
Membership	Process experts, cross functional	Process experts, cross functional
Training	Benchmarking and improvement/planning tools, group dynamics, team management	QI tools, group dynamics, team management
Procedures	Benchmarking steps, 7 meeting steps, facilitator/adviser assistance	Process improvement model, 7 meeting steps, facilitator assistance
Group Dynamics	Common stages of development plus special closing stage; focus on dynamics	Common stages of development plus special closing stage; focus on dynamics
Duration	*Ad hoc*	*Ad hoc*

Purpose

The benchmarking team is established to find, adapt, and implement best practices in order to achieve breakthrough performance. The first stage in fulfilling this purpose is to study and understand exactly how the process operates currently. Next the team measures performance of the process and explains, with supporting data, what variables determine that performance. The third stage toward fulfillment of purpose is for the team to study and understand the performance and the process—that is, the practices—of its "best-in-class" partner(s). Finally, the team must adapt and implement these best practices in order to ensure success in its unique culture and satisfaction among its own customers.

Leadership

Leadership of the benchmarking team is determined on the basis of process ownership and several other criteria, including availability of an individual to participate in the study, as described in chapter 6. Whether or not the actual or "virtual" owner of the process leads the team, she or he is directly involved, either as co-leader or through regular consultation. Selection of a leader on the basis of ownership is crucial because it reinforces the importance of the process as the focus of the benchmarking effort. Further, appropriate choice in leadership can facilitate implementation of improvements discovered by the team if the process owner/leader can influence directly the action to be taken. Practically speaking, this will nearly always imply that the leader is chosen from the manager ranks of the organization.

Membership

Team members, of course, are drawn from the ranks of those who know and operate the process; usually they represent multiple departments. Direct familiarity with the subtleties and nuances of the process under study enables members not only to understand the current process but to be more adept in incorporating the best practices uncovered. This means that even at the collaborative level the benchmarking team cannot consist exclusively of managers who, by virtue of their positions, do not have firsthand knowledge of process operations. Nonetheless, because managers have a big-picture view of the process and its implications—and therefore ownership—their representation on the team is necessary.

Training

Because benchmarking, like CQI generally, represents a paradigm shift in how the organization improves, teams must have the requisite know-how and process-specific skills. Therefore, teams receive extensive training, not just in a general benchmarking methodology or in process analysis, but in methods and tools of team management and group dynamics. Specific areas of knowledge and the tools needed to do benchmarking effectively are discussed later in this chapter.

Procedure

As a discipline, benchmarking is based on the scientific method and on the premise of continual improvement. Therefore, teams utilize procedures that reflect this grounding. As made clear in this book, the collaborative benchmarking model is an adaptation of Shewhart's PDCA cycle; steps in the model as adapted herein provide a framework that guides teams through the procedures. For example, a step-by-step meeting methodology (described later in this chapter) may be used to assist in a successful outcome. Team management tools such as brainstorming, decision matrixes, and consensus ensure optimal contribution and ownership by members. Each meeting includes an evaluation of the meeting process to facilitate improvement in teamwork and use of the benchmarking methods. These procedure-oriented activities reinforce the scientific method on which benchmarking is based.

Group Dynamics

The team deliberately accesses group dynamics rather than leaving this powerful dimension to chance. In learning about or reviewing the developmental stages through which work groups pass (described later in this chapter), members take collective responsibility for their interrelationships and behaviors that affect teamwork. The facilitator/adviser draws on the group dynamic–teamwork dimension to help resolve problems and to provide feedback for improvement.

Duration

By design, benchmarking teams generally are *ad hoc coalitions*, that is, temporary. They end with implementation of the best practices found during the study. In certain situations the team, or some members, might be called back into service—for example if performance data indicate difficulty with holding the gain achieved initially. In this event, they are more likely to act as a typical QI team rather than as a benchmarking team.

Variables in Benchmarking Team Success

Selecting and chartering a benchmarking team in each organization does not automatically ensure the team success. Many variables act together to influence how effective the team, and consequently the benchmarking study, proves to be. Figure 8-2 identifies six key factors that guide successful teamwork. These key areas are summarized in the following subsections.

Team Management

The benchmarking team itself represents a process to be managed, from how it uses time to how it organizes its work. The team must maintain a clear focus on its mission and follow the project road map closely. In addition, the team should establish clear roles, both formal and informal, as discussed in the next section. Meetings will be managed more effectively if the team makes use of a structured process such as the "Seven Meeting Steps" developed by Executive Learning, Inc.:[1]

1. Review the objective for the meeting.
2. Review team meeting roles (leader, recorder, timekeeper, facilitator).
3. Review the agenda items (including method and time allotted for each).
4. Work through the agenda.
5. Review the meeting record (determine what to retain for the next meeting and for the team's "storyboard" or notebook).
6. Determine next steps (in the project) and next meeting agenda.
7. Evaluate the meeting (what went well and what can be improved).

Figure 8-2.   Fishbone Diagram Showing Key Variables in Effective Benchmarking Teams

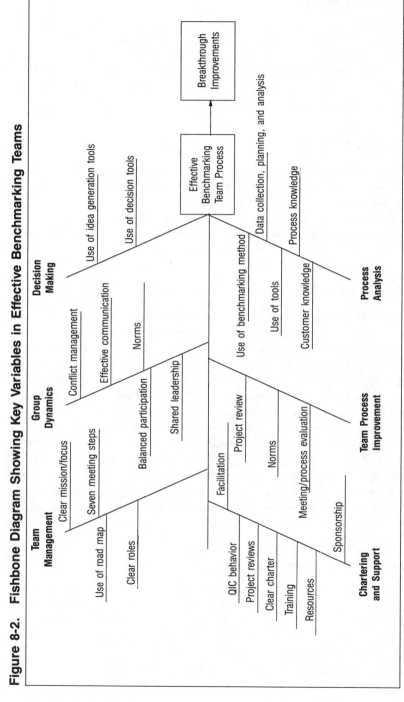

Adapted from: Mosel, D., and Shamp, M. J. Enhancing quality improvement team effectiveness. *Quality Management in Health Care* 1(2):47–57, 1993.

Group Dynamics

Group dynamics are a powerful variable in terms of personal styles and inter-personal relationships that directly affect the team's ability to use benchmark-ing methods and tools. Effective teams develop mutually understood and acceptable norms to guide member behavior to ensure that team "chemistry" is compatible with its mission. Typically, specific norms are established to help the team manage communication and conflict.

Decision Making

Making good use of idea generation tools facilitates both *divergent thinking* (var-ious methods of brainstorming to promote creativity) and *convergent thinking* (the decision matrix, for example, to focus on a limited number of possibili-ties). Decision-making tools, such as multivoting or the decision matrix, assist the team in generating a sense of shared ownership for its decisions, preferably by consensus.

Chartering and Support

Effective chartering and support on the part of the quality council or senior management team in each participating organization is the first rung on the team success ladder. Although a project charter is drawn for and by the col-laborative, the focus here is on how chartering and support for the benchmark-ing team are provided at the organizational level. The quality council first develops a clear mission statement for the team, from which the team derives its direction. As explained in chapter 6, the team charter includes not only the mission but the project goal, identification of team leader and members, a road map delineating how the project will proceed, a time line, and antici-pated budget. Effective support for teams also includes resources (financing and release time to work on the project, for instance) and training (detailed later in this chapter). Finally, quality council support provides for regular reviews of progress with the benchmarking team (also discussed in a later section of this chapter).

Team Process Improvement

Teamwork is a process. As such it is also the focus of improvement. Evaluating each meeting (meeting step 7) provides a regular opportunity for the team to identify strengths and opportunities for improvement in its work. Project review sessions with the quality council are specific occasions for learning how to improve the team's use of both benchmarking and team management methods. (The review session is detailed later in this chapter.)

Process Analysis

Success of the benchmarking effort rests heavily on the team's capacity to analyze work processes, first within its own organization during the internal study, then outside as it examines the practices of external partners. This capacity includes understanding and using benchmarking methods and related tools such as flowcharting and cause-effect analysis, as well as management planning tools such as the affinity diagram or tree diagram. The team must have knowledge of its own work process and of the requirements of customers served by that process. Process analysis requires team proficiency in collecting and interpreting the data needed to quantify process outcomes and explain process variation.

Team Roles

The benchmarking team fills several roles in carrying out its work: leader, member, timekeeper, and recorder. In addition, the special roles of facilitator/adviser and sponsor serve in a support capacity to the team. Individuals in the last two roles generally are not considered team members.

Team Leader

When possible, the team leader is the owner of the process being studied. Chapter 6 defined process ownership and focused on the attributes and selection of the team leader. This subsection emphasizes the role of the process owner/leader in relation to the team. Working closely with the facilitator/adviser, this individual leads team meetings and co-plans with the facilitator each meeting's agenda based on input from individual team members (meeting step 6). During meetings the leader manages the seven-step process described above, while retaining his or her own role as a knowledgeable member of the team. When appropriate, this person shares leadership with other members, for example, when someone else might guide the team in a flowcharting exercise or present a part of the team's report in a review session with the quality council.

The other primary role of the leader is to coordinate the project between meetings, such as directing a data collection effort. The benchmarking team leader represents the team in contacts with the project sponsor or others from the quality council.

Team Member

The team member is an expert in the process chosen for the benchmarking study. Because members work in the process directly, they have firsthand knowledge of its current way of operating. Members contribute this knowledge of the process throughout the project, especially during internal benchmarking and during implementation of best practices identified in the external study. During team meetings, members take the roles of timekeeper and recorder, taking care not to step outside their role as process experts. Between meetings, they may be assigned other tasks, such as collecting performance data on the process being studied.

Timekeeper

The timekeeper monitors the time budgeted for each agenda item in team meetings and reports to the team in a way that facilitates time management. This role is rotated among team members from meeting to meeting.

Recorder

The recorder, another rotated role, involves recording important information such as results of a decision process or data analysis done during team meetings. The recorder is generally the one who will use the flipchart to capture important ideas, analyses, or actions for the team. He or she will also update the team's storyboard or notebook following the meeting.

Facilitator/Adviser

The facilitator/adviser is a specialist in benchmarking and process analysis method and tools, group dynamics and team management, and idea generation and decision-making tools. He or she is not an expert in the process under study but assists the team leader by helping to plan meetings and by giving the leader postmeeting debriefs and feedback on strengths and opportunities for improvement. During meetings, the facilitator supports both leader and team through just-in-time training, by interrupting the team's process to examine its effectiveness, or to offer an alternative method or tool. Facilitators are generally selected from among managerial or professional ranks of the organization, based on criteria established by the quality council (credibility and respect among peers and demonstrated interpersonal and group skills, for example).

Sponsor

The sponsor (the project champion) is usually a member of the quality council to whom the team leader reports. As liaison between the benchmarking team and senior managers of the organization, she or he does not act as a member of the team and usually attends meetings only at the team's request. The sponsor helps maintain priority and visibility of the benchmarking study among members of the quality council. The sponsor plays a very important role in implementation of best practices and/or new processes. For example, this individual's knowledge of organizational priorities and politics can be crucial in helping the team identify and manage resistance to change.

Stages of Team Development

As with any group, benchmarking team dynamics develop through a series of stages which, if left unattended, can slow or even derail progress of the study. When these stages are managed effectively, team progress is actually accelerated. Each developmental stage is characterized by certain team behaviors and needs. The names given these stages (the first four of which names were coined by Barbara Tuckman) reflect the essence of team dynamics at that stage.[2] Figure 8-3 presents a description of the four stages of team development, including for each stage typical characteristics, feelings and behaviors, critical tasks, and pitfalls and solutions. The additional stage of "closing" is also described.[3]

One of the key roles of the benchmarking facilitator/adviser is to observe the developmental dynamics of the team and to assist the team and team leader with management of each stage. The facilitator/adviser does this through just-in-time (JIT) training of the team, planning with the team leader, and through intervention. Just-in-time training occurs at the invitation of the team or leader, or when the facilitator observes the need to interrupt the process for the purpose of teaching. This individual meets with the leader before each team meeting, as described earlier, to help plan the agenda and the use of appropriate methods and tools. In the debriefing session following each meeting, the facilitator and leader evaluate the work of the team and identify improvements to be made. The facilitator/adviser intervenes when the team or leader needs a hand with teamwork issues or with the use of methods and tools. For example, if the team and its leader are unable to resolve a conflict, the facilitator intervenes to offer feedback and engage the team in developing a strategy to deal with the situation. Or if the team begins to use an analytical tool such as a run chart inappropriately, the facilitator's role is to intervene to ensure that the run chart is constructed and interpreted according to proven practice.

Training Requirements

The novice team requires extensive training in benchmarking methodology and possibly in the use of related tools. Managers and staff in organizations that already have CQI experience will need less training in these areas. In both cases, the benchmarking collaborative must ensure that teams receive the training they need. The benchmarking team must be competent in benchmarking methodology, quality planning and redesign, team dynamics, descriptive statistics, process improvement, data collection, and project management (among

Figure 8-3. Stages of Team Development

Stage 1. Forming

- *Characteristics:* Dependence on the leader, need for orientation
- *Feelings and behaviors:* Excitement, uncertainty; superficial, cautious interaction; questions, waiting for direction
- *Critical tasks:* Introductions, inclusion of members; clarification of project charter and structure
- *Pitfalls and solutions:* "Jumping to solutions"—review benchmarking approach/scientific method; low ownership of mission—review of charter, emphasis on payoff to organization and team; uneven inclusion—warmup/team-building exercises, introduction of team members, establish ground rules related to participation

Stage 2. Storming

- *Characteristics:* Conflict, clarification of member roles and styles of charter and benchmarking methods
- *Feelings and behaviors:* Frustration, defensiveness; aggression/withdrawal; engagement
- *Critical tasks:* Accepting differences, sharing influence, clarifying roles and project/meeting methods
- *Pitfalls and solutions:* Hidden conflict—identify and sanction differences; dominant behaviors—structured participation, consensus decisions on ground rules/methods; resistance to approach or to others' ideas—inclusion, inquire to understand, consensus

Stage 3. Norming

- *Characteristics:* Team cohesion, trust, open exchange
- *Feelings and behaviors:* Positive regard, comfort; acceptance, friendliness, sharing information, inquiry, feedback
- *Critical tasks:* Development of team norms and team spirit (cohesion)
- *Pitfalls and solutions:* Conflict avoidance—clear norms/ground rules regarding value of conflict/diversity; drift from focus—balance attention to agenda/project and teamwork; "groupthink"—structure participation, focus on differences, test consensus

Stage 4. Performing

- *Characteristics:* Shared leadership, collaboration, productive work
- *Feelings and behaviors:* Mutual respect, satisfaction, confidence; conflict management; flexible use of method/tools
- *Critical tasks:* Sharing leadership, effective application of method, progress review with quality council, completion of project, learning from experience
- *Pitfalls and solutions:* Directive leadership/facilitation—planned reduction of leader/facilitator direction as team competence increases

Stage 5. Closing

- *Characteristics:* Drawing to completion, celebration
- *Feelings and behaviors:* Pride, mix of sadness and satisfaction; ambivalence, avoidance
- *Critical tasks:* Documentation of project success, transfer of learning, final progress review, recognition/celebration
- *Pitfalls and solutions:* Avoidance of closure—plan for disbanding team and addressing mixed feelings: project "failure"—emphasize lessons learned and their application to next iteration of study, help team manage feelings

others). (See figure 8-4, which summarizes knowledge areas and the groups for whom they are appropriate.) Other key groups in the collaborative (key decision makers and guidance team, for example) will benefit from training to fulfill their support roles in the study.

The basic knowledge necessary for success with collaborative benchmarking is gained through one or more of the following methods: specialized courses or programs (which include content drawn from the areas in figure 8-4), a mentor/teacher (usually an external expert), self-study (reading and seminars or conferences), or practice (use of PDSA cycle). Although a combination of all four is optimal, at least a combination of specialized courses and practice is recommended. In the organization with strong CQI experience, it may only be necessary to provide a two- or three-day introduction to benchmarking. Otherwise, additional education in CQI methods may be necessary to ensure a successful benchmarking experience.

Beyond the knowledge of benchmarking needed as a foundation for a successful study, specific tools are necessary, at least for the benchmarking teams.

Figure 8-4. Areas of Knowledge for Groups in the Collaborative

Area of Knowledge	Group				
	KD	GT	QC	BT	F/A
Benchmarking	✔	✔	✔	✔	✔
Quality planning and redesign		✔		✔	✔
Team dynamics		✔		✔	✔
Facilitating teams					✔
Quality function deployment		✔			✔
Descriptive statistics		✔	✔	✔	✔
Systems thinking	✔	✔	✔		✔
Process improvement	✔	✔	✔	✔	✔
Data collection	✔	✔	✔	✔	✔
Project management		✔	✔	✔	✔
JIT training					✔
Information networking, research		✔			✔

Key to Abbreviations: KD = key decision makers BT = benchmarking team
GT = guidance team F/A = facilitator/adviser
QC = quality council

Optimally, the other key groups in the collaborative will learn the tools as well. Generally, tools are taught "just in time" to the benchmarking team in order to save time and provide for immediate application. Figure 8-5 lists tools and stage(s) in the benchmarking project most appropriate for their use. Whereas any of the tools may be used in a benchmarking study, those shown in bold— such as the seven meeting steps, run charts, and the previsit and postvisit checklists—are used in nearly every project.

Teamwork as a Process for Organizational Learning

As already stated, the benchmarking collaborative undertakes benchmarking for the immediate purpose of learning about, adapting, and implementing best practices to achieve breakthrough performance in key work processes. The longer-term reason is to enhance the organization's capacity for learning. Each step of the study is an opportunity to learn about teamwork, especially across disciplines and departments. It is also an opportunity to learn about learning—about how to accumulate knowledge of customers, processes, and ways of organizing work.

At one level organizational learning is about the use of methods and tools which, through practice, become integrated and accessible for future use. At a deeper level it involves a paradigm shift in understanding about what organizations can become—learning collectives in which all stakeholders pool their knowledge for the benefit of those they serve. When organizations begin to learn on this level, they lay the groundwork for evolving into an ever-improving, learning-based culture.

The benchmarking team is a focal point for organizational learning. The project review sessions are a primary way of making lessons from the team's experience accessible to senior management and to the rest of the organization. How the project review is conducted, then, is crucial in facilitating the organizational learning process. A number of variables have impact on the effectiveness of the review meeting.

Regular Review

The quality council should review the benchmarking team's progress at regular and appropriate intervals during the internal study. Key decision makers should regularly review the work of the collaborative team during external benchmarking. Building review sessions into the project road map ensures that these learning opportunities are treated as a priority and not left to chance.

Preparation of the Council and the Collaborative

Reviewers need to be familiar with both the project and the benchmarking process and to understand that the purpose of review is to learn—both about

Figure 8-5. Tools Used in Each Benchmarking Phase

Tool/Method	Phase			
	1: ST	2: EC	3: IS	4: ES
Critical Pathways			•	•
7 Meeting Steps	•	•	•	•
Decision Matrix	•	•	•	•
Road Map (Gantt chart)		•	•	•
Team Charter	•	•	•	•
PDSA		•	•	•
Consensus	•	•	•	•
Spider Diagram		•	•	•
Affinity Diagram		•	•	•
Activity Network Diagram		•	•	•
Brainstorming	•	•	•	•
Cause–Effect (Ishikawa) Diagram			•	•
Control Charts			•	•
Force-Field Analysis		•	•	•
Interrelationship Digraph			•	•
Multivoting	•	•	•	•
Pareto Diagram			•	•
Previsit Checklist				•
Postvisit Checklist				•
Prioritization Matrixes			•	•
Process Decision Program Chart (PDPC)			•	•
Selection Matrix	•	•	•	•
Tree Diagram		•	•	•
Xerox "Z" Chart			•	•
Run Chart			•	•
Flowchart	•		•	•
Histogram			•	•
Scatter Diagram			•	•

Key to Abbreviations: ST = select topic   IS = internal study
EC = establish collaborative   ES = external study

Note: Most frequently used tools/methods are shown in **boldface type.**

project progress and about what the teams have learned about the methods and tools they are using. The council and the collaborative must model critical behaviors such as attention to presenters, asking open-ended questions, and focus on data and process. The optimal review setting is conducive to a feeling of safety (free of criticism and blame), a tone that is set by senior managers. This means that even when a team is unable to report progress or when a project fails to achieve its goals, the review session places attention on lessons learned about how to improve the benchmarking process rather than on fault finding.

Preparation of the Team

The benchmarking team contributes to a productive review session in several ways. Keeping the record ("storyboard" or project notebook) of the project current is fundamental and means that the team is able to use existing documentation in the review session. Following a standard format in presenting the report facilitates understanding of the team's progress; the PDSA cycle is an excellent framework for reporting during the internal or external study. Rehearsing the presentation is always good advice but is especially useful in anticipating key questions and the most informative ways to respond. Generally, the presentation part of the review session should not exceed 20 to 30 minutes, with additional time allotted for discussion. The authors recommend that teams report *as teams*, so that the review session benefits from multiple perspectives and as a way of recognizing team members. Assigning roles to team members ensures that the presentation flows smoothly. Finally, it is critical that teams identify and communicate lessons learned, not only about the process(es) they are studying, but also about methods, tools, and teamwork.

Best Practices in Teamwork and Organizational Learning

Few health care organizations have mastered the discipline of learning from the experience of teams, either in benchmarking or in quality improvement generally. Following are some examples of organizational "best practices":

- *Parkview Episcopal Medical Center, Pueblo, Colorado,* conducts twice-monthly Quality Forums in which quality improvement teams report on their learning. These all-day sessions are led by the CEO and are open not only to management but to anyone in the organization.
- *Evangelical Health System, Oakbrook, Illinois,* sponsors systemwide quality fairs to focus on improvement successes. The events feature a strong emphasis on learning from experience in the quality journey.

Resources

Listing all resources available to support learning about benchmarking teams and quality improvement teams is unrealistic given the limitations imposed here. However, the following selections may prove helpful.

- *Quality Management in Health Care.* Aspen Publishing (Silver Spring, Maryland). Each issue includes a review on the use of a quality improvement tool.
- The Quality Publication series. AT&T Customer Information Center (Indianapolis, Indiana). Includes books on quality technology and tools as well as quality management and systems. One of the most complete and helpful collections the authors have found.
- Executive Learning, Inc. (Brentwood, Tennessee). Book and series of videotapes on quality improvement and teamwork methods and tools.
- GOAL/QPC. Books and videotapes on the seven quality control tools and the seven management and planning tools, including the well-known Memory Jogger series.
- Leebov, W., and Ersoz, C. J. *The Health Care Manager's Guide to Continuous Quality Improvement.* Chicago: American Hospital Publishing, 1991.
- *The Systems Thinker.* Pegasus Communications (Cambridge, Massachusetts).
- Plsek, P., and Onnias, A. Quality Improvement Tools. Juran Institute.
- Scholtes, P. *The Team Handbook: How to Use Teams to Improve Quality.* Madison, WI: Joiner Associates, 1988.

Summary

Teams are the vehicle through which benchmarking is accomplished. Effectively managed, teams not only accomplish their immediate goal of finding and implementing best practices, but serve as a powerful source of organizational learning. Numerous variables contribute to successful teamwork, from chartering and support for the team on the part of the quality council to the application of process analysis methods. The benchmarking team experience is a powerful source of learning, not only to achieve breakthrough performance but to facilitate transformation of the organization.

Putting These Ideas to Work

Objective

Assess the readiness of your organization to support and learn from benchmarking teams.

Approach

1. How effective has your organization been in learning from teams in the past?

Rate your learning on the following criteria on a scale of 1 to 5 (1 = rarely, 5 = regularly); then plot the numbers on the team learning assessment presented in figure 8-6.

- *Teams:* To what extent does your organization make use of teams to improve work processes?
- *Charter:* Do teams receive clear, focused project charters?
- *Methods:* Are teams provided with systematic methods for improvement and team management?
- *Training:* Do teams receive orientation to projects and methods, as well as just-in-time training during projects?
- *Facilitation:* Are trained facilitators (advisers) assigned to work with teams?
- *Review:* Are projects reviewed regularly in a learning-oriented way by the quality council or senior management?
- *Lessons:* Are lessons learned from teamwork identified and communicated to managers and other teams?

2. Based on your assessment, what are the most important gaps in the readiness of your organization to make optimal use of benchmarking teams as opportunities for learning?
3. What action will you plan to take to close these gaps?

Figure 8-6. Team Learning Assessment

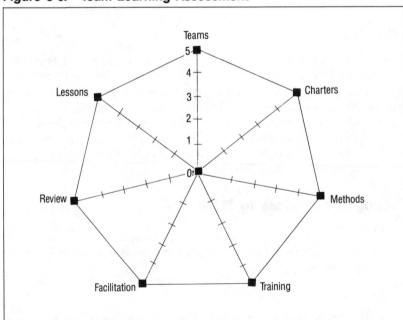

References

1. *Continual Improvement Handbook: A Quick Reference Guide for Tools and Concepts, Healthcare Version.* Brentwood, TN: Executive Learning, 1993.

2. Tuckman, B. Developmental sequence in small groups. *Psychological Bulletin* 63:384–399, 1965.

3. Mosel, D., and Shamp, M. J. Enhancing quality improvement team effectiveness. *Quality Management in Health Care* 1(2):47–57, 1993.

Part Three

Conclusions

Chapter Nine

Lessons Learned and Future Applications

Introduction

The purpose of the benchmarking journey is to improve organizational performance by achieving breakthroughs in a process important to customers. As demonstrated in this text, the collaborative model for benchmarking is a powerful way for health care organizations to achieve that breakthrough performance. The model provides a group approach for organizations to learn collectively and more effectively than as individual entities. This chapter provides some insights into pitfalls to avoid, comments on challenges faced within the collaborative, and speculation about the future application of benchmarking in health care.

The Collaborative Model for Benchmarking in Health Care Organizations

Figure 9-1 summarizes four phases of the collaborative model for benchmarking in health care organizations: selecting the project, establishing the benchmarking collaborative, conducting the internal study, conducting the external study with partners outside the collaborative. The following sections present some of the challenges and pitfalls inherent in each phase of the cycle.

Select the Project

A hazard that befalls most organizations in this phase is *selecting the wrong project.* This can occur if an organization picks a project before determining the criteria for selection. Consequences of inadequate study topics can be limited payoff, a study that is nothing more than someone's pet project, or a project that when completed fails to achieve breakthrough improvement. In either case the organization has invested its limited resources only to become disenchanted with benchmarking as a discipline.

Figure 9-1.   A Collaborative Model for Benchmarking in Health Care

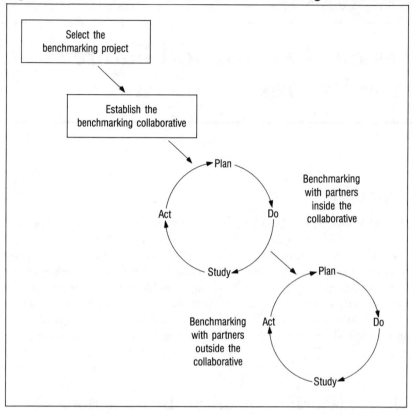

Poor project selection can be avoided by observing the strict guidelines. First, define the conditions proposed projects must meet to be selected as candidates for benchmarking. Second, use these conditions to screen proposed projects routinely. Third, acknowledge a project champion, perhaps a senior leader in the organization who personally sponsors the project. Collectively, these actions help avoid the pitfall of selecting the wrong project.

Establish the Collaborative

Several obstacles can occur within this phase of the collaborative model. These range from misidentifying participants and key decision makers, to inadequate selling of the idea, to poor communication. These and other obstacles discussed below can be overcome, given adequate preparation and persistence on the part of key players.

Misidentifying Potential Participants

The sponsoring organization may make the mistake of identifying only those other organizations with which it has some affinity. Doing so may speed formation of the collaborative but at the risk of restricting the learning that can occur. Organizations are encouraged to examine widely the pool of potential participants for the collaborative, the approach referred to by Spendolini as "thinking out of the box."[1] This especially applies to organizations that do not belong to a health care system. Stand-alone organizations face the challenge of establishing a collaborative with sufficient diversity to provide opportunities for learning. This requires thinking as broadly as possible about internal partners.

Misidentifying Key Decision Makers

Picking the wrong people to make decisions can be avoided by gaining conviction from the top-level managers of participating organizations. The chief executive officer and other senior leaders, for example, must acknowledge the effort and commit to participation. The sponsoring organization must avoid working only with functional managers and go directly to the top of the organization to build legitimacy for participation.

Presenting a Case Inadequately

The sponsoring organization and the project champion may fail to present a strong enough case for the proposed study to warrant participation. This happens frequently because project sponsors are so committed to the project they do not see it objectively. The sponsoring organization can help build a stronger case by critiquing presentations before they are made to potential participants. Critiques allow for improvements in the presentations, building in more objective rationale for participation that is bolstered by good support data.

Defining a Focus Poorly

The project charter should be a concise mission statement, defining the purpose of the collaborative. The group can avoid becoming mired in endless discussion of purpose and mission by focusing on the benchmarking project and the reasons it was selected. Comparing the following two project charters exemplifies this point:

- Identify, adapt, and implement improvements in the inpatient elective admitting process that result in decreased waits for patients, reduced process costs, and increased patient and physician satisfaction.
- Improve the through-put of the admissions process.

The first statement provides significantly more direction and focus for the project. It defines the scope and scale of the effort. It also embodies the rationale for the project and provides definitive measures of project effectiveness.

Miscommunicating Ground Rules

A large collaborative (more than a dozen participants) may wish to set up a guidance team to handle the details of proceeding with the approach. The collaborative can avoid communication problems that may arise between the collaborative and the guidance team by setting up basic ground rules. Examples include sharing meeting minutes within two days of a meeting or establishing common meetings between the two groups on a recurring basis. Once established, these ground rules dictate how the two groups will operate and relate.

Misallocating Time Requirements

Forming a benchmarking collaborative takes longer than one ever plans. Participants can move the effort along by remaining in frequent contact with one another. This is particularly true of those organizations that waver over participation. In addition, frequent standing meetings within the sponsoring organization help maintain momentum until the collaborative is launched.

Conduct the Project Internally

Following are five of the most common pitfalls that occur in this phase of benchmarking. Some suggested ways to avoid them are provided.

Misunderstanding the Internal Process before Engaging Others

This is the most significant pitfall encountered by benchmarking organizations in this phase. It results in failure to discern the important key output characteristics and key process variables, which in turn causes benchmarking teams and the collaborative to focus on the wrong practices. Fortunately, this can be avoided by taking steps to understand and analyze one's own process by identifying the KOCs and KPVs fully. Teams accomplish this by using the proper tools—flowcharting, cause-effect diagrams, and tree diagrams.

Compromising the Scope of the Project

Benchmarking teams often allow the scope of the project to exceed the bounds originally drawn. For example, a team that allows a project to expand from examining employee benefits costs to exploring *all* labor costs obscures the study's intent and thus benchmarking outcomes. Teams can avoid this pitfall by returning to the charter statement during times of uncertainty or contacting the guidance team or benchmarking collaborative for clarity.

Overburdening the Data Collection Process

Benchmarking teams sometimes make data collection unnecessarily complicated and onerous. A large proportion of data collection forms returned incomplete should be a tipoff to this pitfall. This barrier can be overcome by simplifying data collection—reducing the volume of data needed or the period for which data are collected. Only data relevant to the team charter need be collected.

Failing to Search for Internal Best Practices

Often benchmarkers fail to recognize that they can learn from others performing better than they do. One question should be at the forefront of every collaborative effort: "What can be learned from every step in the collaborative model?"

Underestimating the Time Involved

Again, time cannot be downplayed because planning and coordination among participants may take longer than expected. Facility initiatives compete for attention on the managerial agenda, and the benchmarking teams and collaborative can address this issue by allowing extra time when developing the work plan for the internal study phase. A second way to circumvent time miscalculations is to communicate regularly with the leaders in participating organizations.

Conduct the Project Externally

This phase often includes the most complicated steps (researching outside candidates, for example). Therefore, any number of errors can occur during the work of the collaborative.

Failing to Clarify Generic Questions

Posing questions that lack focus can be avoided by returning to knowledge the collaborative already has and examining known gaps in performance of the process. The team must look at its knowledge of customers and how well it understands key output characteristics and key process variables. Doing so helps clarify the questions to be addressed and provide focus. It also allows the collaborative to reinforce its understanding of members' processes, which may lead to further insights for improvement.

Picking the Wrong Partner

Because benefits derived from benchmarking depend in large part on which partners the collaborative selects, picking the wrong partners can prove just as devastating as in phase 2, forming the collaborative. As indicated in chapter 7, focused research using a broad range of resources helps ensure picking the right partners, that is, those that will contribute to learning and improved performance. To expand the search for potential partners, the collaborative must think about this study project and its process in the broadest possible terms, or think generically. Doing so allows the search to reach different secondary and primary sources to identify potential external partners. This broadens the chance to uncover partners that provide wider opportunity for breakthrough improvement.

Another way to avoid picking the wrong partner is to recognize the need for multiple partners. It is unlikely that any one partner can provide all the best practices and supporting enablers the collaborative seeks. Therefore, the collaborative must prepare for dealing with several benchmarking partners simultaneously.

Failing to Develop Specific Questions and Interview Guides

Questionnaires and interview guides must be specific enough to obtain the information required from benchmarking partners. Often these instruments lack the focus necessary to uncover the detailed data from partners required to identify best practices and enablers. The collaborative can overcome this difficulty by structuring their questionnaires and interview guides with three objectives in mind: focusing on performance gaps, paying attention to customer requirements, and learning more about the benchmarking partners' process performance measures. Developing a hierarchy of contingency questions also helps focus discussion. This hierarchy of questions can be constructed using a tree diagram to ensure continuity of the line of inquiry.

Mishandling Site Visits

Conducting site visits presents a challenge to some benchmarkers inexperienced with this process. Protocols created by professional organizations involved with benchmarking ease the planning and scheduling, confirmation, communication, and general coordination that go into a site visit. The International Benchmarking Clearinghouse of the American Productivity & Quality Center has published a code of conduct to help guide this step. The code is presented in figure 5-7 (p. 90) and other sample protocols are presented in figures throughout chapter 7.

Misaligning Performance and Practice

Benchmarking partners best understand the link between their outstanding performance and the practices that drive it. Therefore they are best suited to help the collaborative understand the relationship between performance and best practices identified. Once the collaborative understands this relationship, it must find ways to adapt these practices to their respective settings. Before this can happen, however, the participants must know their own processes and customer requirements. One technique for establishing the proper practice-performance relationship is to work backward from the desired result through the process and the practices that produce that result. Starting with the "end" in mind, participants can create improved means (processes) that incorporate the practices learned and adapted from benchmarking partners.

Five-Stage Life Cycle of a Collaborative

The collaborative will encounter challenges and pitfalls along the journey that occur outside the four phases of the benchmarking model. Some of these danger zones relate to the collaborative; some to the members that compose it.

While focusing on a project, the collaborative has a limited scope and lifespan. This may cause each member's senior management to view it as a "special" project. By definition, special projects have life-cycle stages of their own, not unlike the stages of team development. Those stages of team development include: forming, storming, norming, performing, and closing.[2] Some potential pitfalls that can occur in these stages are discussed below.

Forming

Forming represents the orientation and initiation stage of the collaborative and its effort. Potential pitfalls during this stage are the basis for the discussion of phase 2, establishing the collaborative (chapter 5). These include identifying potential participants or key decision makers incorrectly; presenting an insufficient case for the project; failing to establish a clear focus; confusing communications between the collaborative and the guidance team; and underestimating the amount of time required to form the collaborative.

Storming

Storming, the stage during which dissatisfaction and disruptive behaviors occur, may manifest itself in many ways. Some organizations may dispute the approach; others may become anxious about the time taken by the activities of the collaborative; still others may be concerned about the time lapse before results are produced. These are normal reactions to excursions into uncharted territory. The collaborative can maintain focus and momentum by dealing with each issue as it occurs and focusing members on the original proposal and work plan.

If the benchmarking effort represents a special project to many participants, other more immediate and pressing issues may challenge it for attention and resources. This often happens when senior leaders of participating organizations do not receive enough communications about the effort and its status. The collaborative can circumvent this reaction by ensuring frequent and regular communication with senior leaders—as can written or verbal monthly reports to key stakeholders on benchmarking project successes. The focus of communication should be on actions taken by the collaborative and its participants to accomplish the group's mission.

Another example of storming behavior is for a participant to quit the project. This may happen at any time but is most likely to occur after the internal benchmarking phase. Several reasons account for this behavior: The organization improved its performance through learning attained in this cycle; initiatives within the departing organization compete for the resources previously dedicated to the benchmarking effort; or the organization fails to see additional payoff in continuing. Depending on the size of the collaborative, a departure could have devastating effects, anywhere from starting a rash of departures, thus destroying the entire collaborative effort, to the collaborative's losing a member that might have contributed additional learning. Either way, the collaborative could lose opportunity for breakthrough.

The collaborative must strive to maintain participation through all phases of the effort by engaging in frequent and regular contact with the representatives from participating facilities. The guidance team uses these communications to assess commitment to the project and the likelihood of continued participation. This allows for early detection of potential departures. Again, the guidance team's communication must focus on the group mission, the work plan and time frame agreed on, and the actions taken to date that lead to improved organizational performance.

Norming

Norming occurs once teams have begun to deal with conflict successfully and to develop trust among group members. The risk here is "groupthink" due to this new-found cohesion. Rather than risk conflict, team members agree with issues presented. This may occur when members privately disagree with the issue but are unwilling to risk revisiting storming.

The group can test for consensus repeatedly to lessen this risk, but doing so requires each participant to voice concerns about the issue under discussion. In addition, the group must be aware of, and sensitive to, the implications of norming.

Performing

Performing is the stage in the collaborative's life cycle at which interdependence among members occurs and results in productive work. The risk facing the group at this stage is the rush to completion. That is, some members, having worked through the previous stages, may just want to finish the effort and turn their attention elsewhere.

This rushing-through behavior can be avoided by reminding the group of its charter. The group also may utilize structured meetings and problem-solving skills to ensure that all issues are considered before focusing on any one solution.

Closing

The collaborative was formed to accomplish a specific task within a given time. Upon completing that task it should adjourn. The collaborative, however, might have trouble achieving closure on the project, or participants may choose to start another project together, using the collaborative model. Either way, the collaborative must achieve closure by ending its role with the *current* project, perhaps by reconvening to assess satisfaction with the degree of implementation and adaptation of best practices. However, actual implementation lies with the individual participants, not with the collaborative. Therefore, the collaborative must determine an end point for its effort on the current project.

Toward this end the collaborative drafts a report of its actions, the lessons learned, and improvements planned by participants. The section on lessons learned incorporates not only the best practices uncovered for adaptation into participants' processes, but those lessons learned about how to better function in a collaborative model. These lessons on improved functioning benefit all participants as they move toward other collaborative ventures, whether benchmarking projects or other cooperative activities.

Projections for Benchmarking in Health Care

The health care industry is in the midst of change as laid out in chapter 2 of this text. Providers are buffeted by forces from a myriad of sources that challenge providers to seek performance breakthrough improvements. The collaborative model for benchmarking offers a vehicle for achieving these breakthroughs more rapidly by identifying best practices to adapt—but only if planners apply the methodology. Many health care benchmarking projects continue to focus on administrative or support areas. Only recently have studies begun to appear in areas of clinical performance. For example, a monthly newsletter now dedicates itself to identifying and promoting exemplary performance, describing administrative, support, and clinical projects.[3] A review of the newsletter's first four issues reveals that the number of benchmarking studies examined split evenly between clinical and support topics.

Proponents of health care reform envision a system that is much more data and outcomes driven. Benchmarking can play a critical role in such a system by improving organizational and system performance. Daniel Lorence, quality improvement manager at the American Medical Association, identified 10 areas in which health care organizations can apply benchmarking:[4]

1. Health outcomes
2. Federal electronic data interchange
3. Accreditation standards
4. Remote monitoring
5. Health networks
6. Pharmacy databases
7. Practice parameters
8. Utilization summaries
9. Health insurance claims
10. Patient surveys

These multiple areas speak to the widespread applicability of benchmarking in health care. As health care organizations face increased demands for greater changes, benchmarking will likely come into greater use.

Despite its increased application, however, benchmarking still raises some concerns about its possible misuse. Figure 9-2 displays a continuum of process management that should help alleviate this concern. Managing processes proceeds from work simplification at the departmental level, focusing on tasks and activities, an approach that represents the most rudimentary way to manage

Figure 9-2.   Approaches to Managing Processes

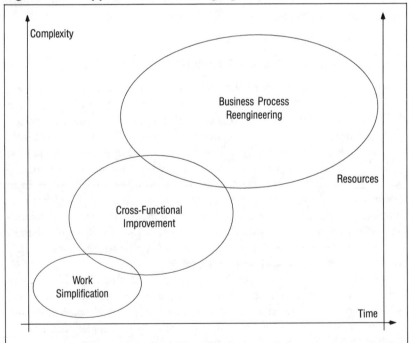

processes. Organizations achieve the next level of maturation in managing processes by working with cross-functional improvement teams, which examine processes that operate across departmental lines. On yet a higher level, organizations may engage in business process reengineering. This level of process management entails design of a new process to meet customer requirements, recognizing that the current process cannot be improved to the degree necessary to meet those needs.

Although benchmarking applies within this construct of process management—for example, within departments to achieve work simplification—it may not provide sufficient payoff to warrant the investment. It is also likely that at this level efforts may degenerate to naive data comparison.

Within the context of cross-functional improvement teams, benchmarking's proper application depends on the scope of the project targeted for improvement. If the team requires improvements of breakthrough proportions, benchmarking may provide the path to discovering such improvements.

At the reengineering level benchmarking projects may apply at two levels. First, benchmarking may help identify and legitimize establishing goals that are orders of magnitude better than current performance. The power of this action cannot be understated. Identifying others' current performance that far exceeds one's own provides a strong impetus for improvement within. Second, benchmarking applied to reengineering projects allows teams to identify best practices to adapt to the design of a new process. As more reengineering occurs within health care organizations, benchmarking performed in support of those efforts will increase. Given that true reengineering projects focus on issues of more strategic importance, benchmarking fits well within such efforts.

Application of Collaborative Models in Other Areas

One lesson learned from using the collaborative benchmarking model is how applicable the model's underlying philosophy of mutual cooperation is to other types of projects. The advantages of bringing organizations together to conduct projects in a cooperative manner cross methodological borders.

The collaborative structure for project design, with this underlying philosophy, has been applied to reengineering projects, one of which involved designing subacute care services. Three long-term care organizations, located in three different states, came together to create new systems of care in anticipation of changing regulatory requirements and growing market factors for subacute services. Benchmarking played a role in the project by identifying existing prototypes for best practices.

The inherent philosophy and structure of the collaborative model also has been applied to services for developmentally disabled persons. Eight independent service agencies across two regions within a state formed a collaborative to design a client-defined, outcomes-based, team planning process for service delivery. Although benchmarking is unlikely to play a large role in this effort, the collaborative approach to resolving problems applies.

A Caution to Benchmarking Proponents

A final caution about the future of benchmarking: Approaches to solving management problems exhibit a life cycle of their own.[5] They come into favor, they fall out of favor. (See figure 9-3.) The cycle begins when current approaches to problem solving fail. This *deficiency* leads to discovery of a new methodology. During the *discovery* stage, the new methodology solves the problems to which it is applied effectively. In the ensuing stage, practitioners are *euphoric* due to the results of early application of the approach. Because these applications worked so well, the methodology gets applied widely—often in instances where other methodologies would be more suitable. Misapplication leads to less-than-expected outcomes, which in turn leads to *derision* for the approach rather than examination of its appropriate use. This denouncement causes users to *abandon* the approach in search for the next management theory.

Those who practice benchmarking in health care organizations must treat the approach for what it is—a methodology for helping organizations achieve breakthrough improvements in performance. Benchmarking represents one

Figure 9-3.   The Life Cycle of a Management Theory

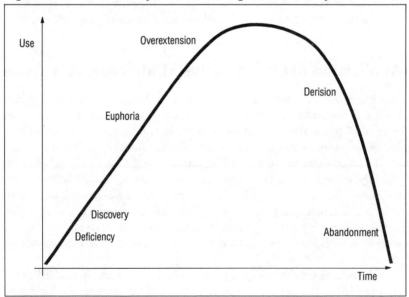

approach toward this end, not the only one. To be used effectively, it must be applied in concert with other process management methodologies.

Summary

The collaborative model for benchmarking in health care offers a powerful, cost-effective way to learn best practices. In that the learning occurs in a cooperative model, both risk and cost to participants are shared. Furthermore, learning occurs at two levels, within and outside the collaborative; thus, the model offers broader horizons from which to gain insights into best practices. The approach builds bridges between participants—both members of the collaborative and outside benchmarking partners—that set foundations for future collaboration, learning, and opportunities for breakthrough improvements. All these work to create healthier communities served.

References

1. Spendolini, M. J. *The Benchmarking Book.* New York City: AMACOM, 1992, p. 23.

2. Mosel, D., and Shamp, M. J. Enhancing quality improvement team effectiveness. *Quality Management in Health Care* 1(2):47–57, 1993.

3. *Hospital Benchmarks: The Newsletter of Best Practices* 1(1–4):1–76, Feb.–May 1994.

4. Lorence, D. Benchmarking quality under U.S. health care reform: the next generation. *Quality Progress* 27(4):103–7, Apr. 1994.

5. Rigby, D. The secret history of reengineering. *Planning Review* 21(2):26, Mar./Apr. 1993.

Additional Books of Interest

Service Quality Improvement: The Customer Satisfaction Strategy for Health Care

by Wendy Leebov, Ed.D., and Gail Scott, M.A.

Provides compelling reasons for focusing organizational attention and resources on continuous service improvement. Includes a comprehensive array of concrete tactics to strengthen service excellence. Plus, strategies to tailor programs to your organization.

Catalog No. E99-136107 (must be included when ordering)
1993. 378 pages, 157 figures, bibliography.
$52.00 (AHA members, $42.00)

Clinical Paths: Tools for Outcomes Management

edited by Patrice L. Spath

Here's an opportunity to see how hospitals and other organizations have successfully incorporated clinical paths into their managed care and outcomes management initiatives. This groundbreaking book explores the major strategy issues related to the development and implementation of clinical paths. It is heavily illustrated with examples of actual paths, sample documentation forms, variance-tracking reports, data analysis instruments, and other practical tools that can generate ideas and assist in the development of outcomes management initiatives.

Catalog No. E99-027101 (must be included when ordering)
1994. 288 pages, 101 figures, 3 tables.
$59.95 (AHA members, $49.95)